MARK WATTS is a consultant ophthalmic surgeon at Arrowe Park Hospital, Wirral. He is the author of many medical information products for the public, including 'Your Cataract Operation', a booklet produced for his own patients. As well as having written a textbook on eye disease, he has published over thirty papers in the medical press and *Cataract: What You Need to Know* for Sheldon Press.

Pl
it

R
A
r

C
Ple
ite
on

Po
Po

Overcoming Common Problems Series

Selected titles
A full list of titles is available from Sheldon Press,
36 Causton Street, London SW1P 4ST, and on our website at
www.sheldonpress.co.uk

Assertiveness: Step by Step
Dr Windy Dryden and Daniel Constantinou

Breaking Free
Carolyn Ainscough and Kay Toon

Calm Down
Paul Hauck

Cataract: What You Need to Know
Mark Watts

Cider Vinegar
Margaret Hills

Comfort for Depression
Janet Horwood

Confidence Works
Gladeana McMahon

Coping Successfully with Pain
Neville Shone

Coping Successfully with Panic Attacks
Shirley Trickett

Coping Successfully with Period Problems
Mary-Claire Mason

Coping Successfully with Prostate Cancer
Dr Tom Smith

Coping Successfully with Ulcerative Colitis
Peter Cartwright

Coping Successfully with Your Hiatus Hernia
Dr Tom Smith

Coping Successfully with Your Irritable Bowel
Rosemary Nicol

Coping with Alopecia
Dr Nigel Hunt and Dr Sue McHale

Coping with Anxiety and Depression
Shirley Trickett

Coping with Blushing
Dr Robert Edelmann

Coping with Bowel Cancer
Dr Tom Smith

Coping with Brain Injury
Maggie Rich

Coping with Candida
Shirley Trickett

Coping with Chemotherapy
Dr Terry Priestman

Coping with Childhood Allergies
Jill Eckersley

Coping with Childhood Asthma
Jill Eckersley

Coping with Chronic Fatigue
Trudie Chalder

Coping with Coeliac Disease
Karen Brody

Coping with Cystitis
Caroline Clayton

Coping with Depression and Elation
Patrick McKeon

Coping with Down's Syndrome
Fiona Marshall

Coping with Dyspraxia
Jill Eckersley

Coping with Eating Disorders and Body Image
Christine Craggs-Hinton

Coping with Eczema
Dr Robert Youngson

Coping with Endometriosis
Jo Mears

Coping with Epilepsy
Fiona Marshall and
Dr Pamela Crawford

Coping with Fibroids
Mary-Claire Mason

Coping with Gout
Christine Craggs-Hinton

Coping with Heartburn and Reflux
Dr Tom Smith

Coping with Incontinence
Dr Joan Gomez

Coping with Long-Term Illness
Barbara Baker

Coping with Macular Degeneration
Dr Patricia Gilbert

Coping with the Menopause
Janet Horwood

Overcoming Common Problems Series

Overcoming Common Problems Series

Overcoming Common Problems

Living with Glaucoma

Mark Watts

sheldon PRESS

First published in Great Britain in 2006

Sheldon Press
36 Causton Street
London SW1P 4ST

British Library Cataloguing-in-Publication Data
A catalogue for this book is available from the British Library

ISBN-13: 978–0–85969–963–1
ISBN-10: 0–85969–963–3

1 3 5 7 9 10 8 6 4 2

Typeset by Deltatype Limited, Birkenhead, Merseyside
Printed in Great Britain by
Ashford Colour Press

Contents

Introduction

Glaucoma is one of the most common, treatable conditions, and yet ignorance of its very existence and misconceptions as to its effects are widespread. It is tragic that in the twenty-first century, people are still unnecessarily losing vision for want of a timely diagnosis, and usually simple treatment. Affecting 1 in 200 of the population over the age of 40, glaucoma accounts for more outpatient attendances at eye departments than any other condition. Its effects present a spectrum of severity ranging from complete absence of symptoms to total blindness, which latter outcome is almost always avoidable if diagnosed soon enough.

It is, par excellence, the condition in which awareness of its existence, and a positive approach to treatment, affect the outcome dramatically. Surprisingly, however, in an age when we are becoming increasingly aware of the importance of healthy living, of our bodies and the importance of early diagnosis of disease, glaucoma remains shrouded in a veil of misunderstanding and unawareness. Partly this is due to the enigmatic nature of the condition, which has hidden its secrets even from those scientists who have researched with a vigour afforded to few other diseases. And yet gradually an understanding of glaucoma has evolved, and the last two decades have seen tremendous advances in discovering the fundamental nature of the condition, and ways of treating it.

The aim of this book is to lift the veil of confusion, and to explain in simple terms what glaucoma means in practical terms for those who have it and also their families. Most people with the condition can lead full lives, totally unaffected by it, other than needing to have treatment and attend for periodic checks, but sadly others suffer more serious effects. We shall consider all the common scenarios that may develop through the condition, and how early diagnosis and effective treatments can mitigate its effects.

I have not tried to conceal the uncertainties that remain about glaucoma among scientists and clinicians alike, since these can sometimes be reflected in difficult decisions about diagnosis and treatment. Indeed, some of the current debates about the very nature of glaucoma are interesting in their own right.

Most of glaucoma diagnosis and treatment, however, is straightforward, but requires a basic understanding of the condition to be best able to make the modest lifestyle changes that may be required. It is incumbent upon us all to have at least some awareness of the existence of glaucoma, and ideally some understanding also of the implications of the diagnosis.

The main message that I hope will come through in this text is the importance of early diagnosis and, in turn, how crucial it is to attend for regular eye checks at the optometrist (previously known as an optician) in order to achieve this. In addition, however, reading this book should also give an appreciation that being diagnosed as suffering from glaucoma is not the terrible sentence that some people wrongly believe. It is instead an opportunity to take control of the condition, and prevent loss of vision – an opportunity that is not repeated.

1
What is glaucoma?

Glaucoma is a condition in which the pressure within the eye is raised to such a degree that damage is caused to the nerves in the eye, and loss of vision results. It is an extremely common condition, and although it often conjures up images of blindness and distress, it can usually be treated effectively if diagnosed sufficiently early, and poor outcomes are very much the exception. In the early stages of the disease, there are usually no symptoms at all, and the very gradual progression of loss of the peripheral field of vision is often not noticed until it has significantly advanced. It is indeed this very capricious nature of glaucoma that poses the main challenge to early diagnosis and treatment.

Who gets glaucoma?

Glaucoma is common, and increasingly so with age. Approximately 1 per cent of people in the 40 to 50 age group are affected by glaucoma, while the condition is three times as common in those aged between 70 and 80. Undoubtedly there is a genetic component to the risk of glaucoma. Although quoted figures vary, the presence of glaucoma in a close relative increases the chance of developing the condition by several times. However, it is not (except in some very specific and uncommon types of glaucoma) inherited in a precise, predictable way like some other diseases in which it can be predicted that 1 in 2 or 1 in 4 children of an affected parent will suffer from it. It is best to think of a family history as simply increasing the risk of developing glaucoma. Similarly, there is a higher incidence in certain races (in particular, Afro-Caribbeans), in those

1

who are diabetics, and in those who are short-sighted. Although certain studies have claimed an association with raised blood pressure, it is not clear whether this is related to glaucoma at all. Men and women are equally likely to develop the condition. Although certain risk factors can be identified, it is clearly sensible in such a common condition to take the precaution of screening for the disease anyway as people enter their fifth decade and beyond. We shall consider this important topic in more detail later in the book.

Understanding the evolution and management of glaucoma involves first some consideration of the normal state of the eye, and in particular how the normal pressure in the eye is developed and influenced by different factors.

Pressure in the normal eye

The pressure in the eye is maintained by the inherent stiffness of the outer coating of the eye, the presence of a gel in the back of the eye termed the *vitreous* gel, and the constant production and drainage of *aqueous* fluid in the front one-third of the eye. It is the variation in flow of the aqueous that is the principal determinant of the pressure within the eye, rather as the pressure in a balloon is affected by the volume of air it is inflated with.

Figure 1 illustrates the anatomy of the eye. The interior of the eye can be broadly thought of as comprising three compartments. These are the *anterior* and *posterior chambers*, both of which are in front of the *lens*, and the *vitreous cavity*, which lies behind it, and is filled with the vitreous gel. The anterior chamber is the space between the back of the clear *cornea* through which we see, and the coloured *iris* of the eye, and the posterior chamber is behind the iris, but in front

2

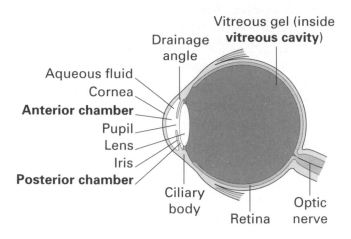

Figure 1 Anatomy of the eye

of the lens. The anterior and posterior chambers communicate through the *pupil*, and they are both filled with watery fluid, termed the aqueous. The aqueous is constantly exchanged by being formed within the posterior chamber and, after flowing through the pupil into the anterior chamber, is then drained away. The production of the aqueous is by a structure termed the *ciliary body*.

This important component of the eye not only has the vital role of producing aqueous, but also supports the lens of the eye, by its attachment to it through fine suspensory filaments. The ciliary body also contains muscles, which contract and relax to control the focusing of the lens. Although this function is not relevant to consideration of aqueous flow, it illustrates the vital roles of the ciliary body. Once the aqueous has flowed into the anterior chamber through the pupil, it then drains through a form of sieve called the *trabecular meshwork,* which is situated in the anterior chamber in the angle between the cornea and the periphery of the iris. This area of the eye is indeed referred to as the *drainage angle*. From the drainage angle, the aqueous is in turn reabsorbed into the bloodstream, via the small veins draining the trabecular meshwork.

Although a somewhat simplistic analogy, I find it helpful to think of this system as being similar to a bath in which the taps (the ciliary body) are on, while the plughole (the trabecular meshwork) remains open. As long as the rate of flow into the bath equals the rate of drainage from it, then the water level (pressure within the eye) remains constant. If the plughole becomes slightly blocked, however, then the level of the water will rise, and indeed the commonest cause of glaucoma is obstruction of the trabecular meshwork. Any imbalance between the flow of aqueous in and out of the eye will lead to a change in the pressure. Although it is normal for the pressure to fluctuate somewhat from day to day, and indeed during the day, a sustained or repeated rise in pressure may lead to nerve damage. Although we shall return to a more detailed study of how different forms of glaucoma can lead to the common endpoint of raised pressure within the eye, let us now consider what the effects of such pressure rises might be.

The effects of raised pressure in the eye

In order to understand a diagnosis of glaucoma and your treatment, it is important to understand the mechanism by which raised pressure damages vision. This is the point at which some uncertainty arises in the understanding of glaucoma, and although the *optic nerve*, which is the site of damage, has been more closely studied than any other single part of the human body, and although glaucoma research can be measured in literally hundreds of thousands of erudite papers and studies, the fundamental mechanism of nerve damage is still not absolutely certain.

It is likely that a number of factors contribute to the death of what are termed *ganglion cells*. These are the vital parts of the optic nerve conduction system, which transmits electrical signals formed by the retina in response to visual stimuli, ultimately to the brain for interpretation as vision. Our current state of understanding is that raised pressure within the eye damages these cells either by direct pressure, or in conjunction with damage to the very delicate blood supply to the nerve, which may either occur independently, or also as a result of the raised pressure. It is known that glaucoma may in some way be genetically caused, and it is probably this genetic predisposition, combined with the raised pressure, that leads to the damage. The pressure may affect the nerve either by reducing further the blood flow to the optic nerve, or possibly by interfering with the flow of nutrients to the nerve. This mechanism, hypothetical as it may be, can be used to explain the apparent paradoxes of those people who have high pressure for many years without ever developing glaucoma damage, and those who develop loss of vision in spite of never developing pressures above 'normal' (so-called *low tension glaucoma*).

The combination of raised pressure and inadequate blood supply to the nerve acts to set off a sequence of events within the cells and their supporting tissues, which leads to their progressive destruction. Harold Quigley, one of the world leaders in glaucoma research, proposed some years ago the model of 'programmed cell death', a hypothesis he supported with experimental animal research, as a mechanism for damage to the optic nerve. We know from direct observation of the optic nerve as it enters the eye, together with microscope

5

studies of eyes with glaucoma, that the supporting connective tissue of the optic nerve as it leaves the back of the eye is gradually eroded in glaucoma. Visualization of this part of the optic nerve termed the *optic nerve head* is one of the three critical parameters for diagnosing and treating glaucoma, the other two being the pressure within the eye and the extent of the field of vision that the eye can perceive.

It is likely that there are many factors that contribute to the loss of nerve function in glaucoma, and these may vary between different people, and different sub-types of glaucoma. If, by definition, we regard glaucoma as a collection of conditions, unified by the common end point of damage to the optic nerve leading to loss of the field of vision, we can then look more precisely at the variety of types of glaucoma that can lead to this.

2
Types of glaucoma

Doctors love to categorize diseases, and in the process give them long, complicated names that seem incomprehensible to those who have not studied them. Although this may seem like an attempt to preserve the mystique of medicine, it can be helpful to break down conditions into sub-groups that have different origins, behaviour or, most importantly, treatments. Glaucoma can be readily subdivided in such a manner, and although the intention of this book is to maintain simplicity and clarity, it is worth looking at the conventional medical classification of glaucoma, to consider the different means by which damage to the optic nerve may develop. Glaucoma, then, is usually divided into the following categories:

Congenital glaucoma

It seems astonishing that a condition that principally affects adults in their latter years, and increasingly so with age, can also affect the newborn baby. Sadly, however, this is the case and, although it is very rare, it is possible for babies to be born with glaucoma. This is known as *congenital glaucoma*. Because the disease presents so early, at a time when normal visual function should still be developing, it often has very serious consequences, resulting sometimes in blindness, even when treated.

The condition usually develops as a result of failure of development of the normal drainage angle. This may be an isolated phenomenon, but often is associated with other abnormalities, either within the eye, or of other organs. We have seen that the effect of raised pressure within the adult eye is damage to the optic nerve, and

7

erosion of the supporting connective tissues around it. In children, whose eyes are still growing, these effects are compounded by a stretching of the cornea and the white connective tissue of the eye termed the *sclera*. This in turn leads to an enlargement of the eye, and eventually damage and scarring of the clear cornea, rather as a balloon might be damaged if it is over-inflated. Although rupture of the eye – as might occur in the balloon that is blown up too much – is rare, the permanent effects of excessive pressure in the formative weeks and months of the eye are serious.

It is a cruel irony that in the early stages of congenital glaucoma, the enlarged cornea caused by the raised pressure may prompt admiring comments from relatives and others attracted by the appealing appearance the eyes may assume. The 'big, bright eyes' admired by Grandmother may turn out to be seriously diseased. It is important, though, to stress that the condition is extremely rare, and the normal attractive eyes of the newborn should not be misdiagnosed as glaucoma!

Children whose eyes are more seriously affected may develop intense light sensitivity, causing them to screw their eyes up tightly, and this discomfort is accompanied by profuse watering. Examination of the cornea in such cases may reveal not only enlargement, but a cloudy, white appearance, indicating waterlogging and swelling through the raised pressure. Effectively the excessive pressure has forced aqueous fluid into the normally relatively dehydrated cornea, overcoming its natural waterproofing properties.

Damage is not isolated to the cornea, however, and the same effects of optic nerve damage that occur in the adult lead to loss of vision in the child also. If the vision is damaged early in life, it is not uncommon for the eyes to wander seemingly randomly, rather than move together in a purposeful manner. This wandering is termed *nystagmus*, and is not unique to glaucoma. Indeed, in the first few weeks of life, there is a tendency for the eyes to move in a rather uncoordinated manner anyway. If glaucoma is present, early treatment is essential to minimize damage to the developing eye.

Juvenile glaucoma

Congenital glaucoma, by definition, is present at birth, even if it takes some months for the diagnosis to become apparent. Some people, however, develop glaucoma at an early age, but not as infants. This type of glaucoma is termed *juvenile glaucoma*, and is used to include those who develop glaucoma up to the age of around 35. It may have strong genetic associations, and certainly the diagnosis should prompt an examination of other family members.

Open angle glaucoma

This is far and away the commonest type of glaucoma, and the one that we shall consider in most detail throughout the book. The term *open angle glaucoma* is used to distinguish it from the much rarer and more dramatic condition of *closed angle glaucoma*, whereby there is a sudden, rapid increase in pressure in the eye due to complete closure of the drainage angle.

In open angle glaucoma, although the drainage angle is obstructed, this blockage is partial, and the rise in pressure is usually gradual and moderate. To refer to our analogy of the bath with the taps on and the plug out, perhaps this is the equivalent of a few hairs blocking up the outflow of the bath, with initially relatively little effect on the level of water.

9

Open angle glaucoma is further subdivided into *primary* and *secondary glaucoma*, depending on whether the angle obstruction is something that just occurs as an isolated phenomenon, or whether it is secondary to some other condition. For example, an eye that has suffered a severe injury may have sustained sufficient damage that the drainage angle is unable to function properly, and the outflow of aqueous is reduced. Similarly, repeated inflammation in the eye, or even the flaking of the normal pigment of the iris and its deposition in the angle, can cause secondary glaucoma.

Other causes of secondary glaucoma include obstruction to the drainage angle by abnormal blood vessels, which can develop in diabetes and other conditions, and also the use of steroid drops in the eye. These are prescribed for a variety of purposes, generally to treat inflammation, but in some predisposed individuals can lead to glaucoma. Usually this reverses when the steroid drops are stopped, but the effects can be permanent.

An unusual form of secondary glaucoma, seen particularly in those of Celtic descent, is termed *pseudo-exfoliative glaucoma*. This condition leads to a flaky deposit on the front surface of the lens, which also can block up the drainage angle. Its significance lies not only in its association with glaucoma, but also with a tendency for the lens bag and its suspensory filaments to be very weak. This can make cataract surgery more hazardous, should it be needed, particularly since the pupil often dilates poorly. *Pigmentary glaucoma* is another type of secondary glaucoma, whereby some of the pigment from the back surface of the iris rubs off and obstructs the aqueous outflow through the angle. Although these seem rather technical details, their recognition by the specialist is important, since they can influence treatment strategies.

Overall, secondary glaucoma is very much less

common than primary glaucoma. The vast majority of cases of glaucoma, then, are of the type called *primary open angle glaucoma*. In reading about glaucoma in medical texts, you will often come across the acronym POAG to refer to this condition, and it is also sometimes known as *chronic simple glaucoma* or CSG. Perhaps it would be better to regard it as ordinary or 'common or garden' glaucoma!

Closed angle glaucoma

This is a relatively rare type of glaucoma, but one that can have dramatic and devastating effects if not diagnosed and treated very promptly. Although most of those with the more common open angle glaucoma have probably had the condition for months or years before it is even diagnosed, *closed angle glaucoma* develops suddenly and can lead to loss of vision within days, or even hours.

While the pressure rise in open angle glaucoma is usually gradual and moderate, the pressure in closed angle glaucoma can rise from normal to two or three times normal pressure within the space of an hour or so, and consequently there are symptoms associated with it. These include pain, blurring, haloes, and even general upset that may include nausea and vomiting can develop.

The disease is so different from the types of glaucoma we have discussed so far that it is really worth thinking of it as a different disease. The unifying feature is, of course, raised pressure leading to nerve damage, but the presentation, effects, and indeed treatment, of closed angle glaucoma are so different to the other types that we shall consider the condition on its own in a separate chapter later in the book.

Low tension glaucoma

It seems something of a contradiction to have a variant of glaucoma in which the pressure, or tension, within the eye is seemingly normal, but this is what *low tension glaucoma* refers to. This is also known as *normal tension glaucoma*. In other words, all the usual features of glaucoma, such as loss of the field of vision and damage to the optic nerve, are seen in the presence of normal pressure within the eye. It is not a common form of glaucoma, and, because the pressure is low or normal, may be difficult to diagnose, since in primary open angle glaucoma it is often the raised pressure that suggests the diagnosis in the first place. In addition, it is possible for pressure on the nerve *behind* the eye to lead to similar findings, necessitating scans of the eye socket and brain sometimes to exclude.

The mechanisms of nerve damage in low tension glaucoma are still unclear, and may be different to those involved in the more common types of glaucoma. It is probably best to consider the condition as being one in which the optic nerve is unduly susceptible to pressure, and suffers the same damage from normal pressure within the eye as would a normal eye with raised pressure. Not only is diagnosis something of a dilemma in this condition, but the treatment also is difficult and controversial. The basic principle of management of most forms of glaucoma is lowering of the pressure within the eye, but in low tension glaucoma it is already normal or low!

3
Diagnosis

Early diagnosis is critical to the management of glaucoma. As we shall see later, treatment is unable to reverse damage that has already occurred, and is confined to preventing or delaying visual loss, hopefully before it has become significant. Since symptoms do not usually present until late in the condition, diagnosis is almost always made either through screening, or at a routine eye examination. Most commonly, this is the one undertaken by an optometrist, and highlights one of the many reasons for attending for regular examinations.

Symptoms

Glaucoma is characterized by its lack of symptoms in the early stages, and sadly this accounts for the majority of cases in which treatment is unsuccessful. Any damage that occurs to the eye is irreversible, and if treatment begins too late because the diagnosis was delayed through this lack of symptoms, then severe visual loss can result. Thankfully, this happens in a minority of cases, but it is important to stress that a lack of any apparent problem does not exclude the diagnosis. The much rarer type of glaucoma called *angle closure glaucoma* is an exception to this rule, and in this condition there are symptoms of blurring and pain, which we shall discuss in more detail in Chapter 8.

We have seen that glaucoma is caused by raised pressure within the eye, but the eye is not sensitive enough to detect such rises unless they are extreme. Although there may well be pain in the eye if the pressure reaches twice or three times the normal level (as it may do in angle closure glaucoma), and particularly if this occurs suddenly, the gradual and more modest rise in pressure seen in the majority of cases of glaucoma is completely without symptoms.

Some people may become aware of loss of field of vision, but by the time this occurs, damage is usually quite advanced. This is partly because the loss of peripheral vision is very gradual, and so is not noticed, and partly because the field of vision of one eye overlaps that of the other eye. This means that one eye might lose significant vision while the other makes up for it. Sometimes it is on covering the stronger eye that this becomes apparent. Other symptoms, such as reduced colour perception, a generalized blurring or difficulty in dim lighting conditions, can be seen in glaucoma, but are more commonly associated with other diseases, and are not a useful indicator of glaucoma.

Generally, there are no symptoms, and while it is usually the person himself or herself who draws attention to more dramatic medical conditions such as heart attack and stomach ulcer, self-diagnosis is very much the exception in glaucoma.

Methods of diagnosis

The three measurable parameters on which a diagnosis of glaucoma can be made are:

1 Intraocular pressure, which means the pressure within the eye.
2 The appearance of the optic nerve within the eye.
3 The assessment of the field of vision.

Rarely is one of these alone conclusive of the diagnosis, and more commonly it is the consideration of the three together that defines the condition and its management. Inevitably, therefore, in the earliest stages of glaucoma there may be some doubt as to the diagnosis if, for example, one of these parameters is abnormal while the others are within acceptable limits. This may lead to some 'false alarms' about the condition, and it is important to stress that the mere suggestion of the diagnosis, or indeed even its confirmation, is no cause for panic. Let us now consider these three assessments in more detail.

Intraocular pressure

We have seen already that the pressure within the eye is a function of the amount of aqueous fluid produced within the eye and the amount drained through the drainage angle at the periphery of the iris. There are a number of ways of measuring this pressure, and it is identification of raised pressure that prompts diagnosis in the vast majority of cases of glaucoma.

Although technological advances constantly produce new refinements of instruments to check pressure, there are just two different basic types of pressure measurement. The first is termed *contact tonometry*, and the other is *non-contact tonometry*. The term *tonometry*, which is common to both, simply means measurement of pressure.

The difference between the two methods is apparent from their names: in *contact* tonometry, the pressure-measuring instrument makes contact with the eye or, more specifically, the cornea of the eye, after it has been numbed with drops. In *non-contact* tonometry, there is no direct contact with the eye, but a puff of air is blown at the eye, and the small indentation caused by it is measured. Traditionally, the contact form is used within hospital practice, while the non-contact form is more commonly used by optometrists. Both are extremely accurate, even though there are periodic discussions within the medical press as to which might be more so!

Contact tonometry

There are a number of variants of the contact technique of pressure measurement, but they all work by measuring the force required to indent the cornea. The most commonly used one is an assessment undertaken at the *slit-lamp*, which is the microscope which an eye specialist or optometrist routinely uses to examine the eye. The person places his chin on a small rest, while the examiner looks at the eye through the eyepiece, which is rather like a pair of binoculars, and gives a highly magnified stereo view of the eye.

In order to measure the pressure using this instrument, drops containing anaesthetic and a yellow dye are first put into the eye. This allows painless contact with the cornea. The person being tested is asked to look directly ahead, as a small, thimble-shaped device attached via a short metal rod to a strain gauge is brought slowly towards the cornea. As it makes gentle contact with the cornea, a small amount of flattening occurs, which displaces the film of yellow drops. The 'thimble' end of the instrument is actually transparent, and the observer can view this displacement through the microscope. The yellow drops glow green when illuminated with the blue light which is used to do this. By adjusting the strain gauge, the examiner can measure the pressure needed to indent the cornea by a certain amount, and this produces a very accurate measurement.

From the perspective of the person being tested, this is a simple, painless procedure, which simply involves looking straight ahead, as a blue light approaches the eye. A variant of this technique uses a hand-held version of the same machine, and yet another device uses a micro strain gauge in the tip of the instrument to give a digital readout of the pressure.

Non-contact tonometry

The non-contact forms of pressure measurement use a puff of air to assess the pressure of the eye, by measuring the amount that the cornea is distorted when a puff of air of fixed pressure is directed at it. Imagine using the same force to push in the outside of two footballs inflated to different pressures. The one that is more firmly inflated will be indented less than the one that is softer, and this is the principle on which non-contact pressure measurements work. The difference is that a puff of air of fixed pressure is used rather than your thumb!

The advantage of this technique over contact ones is that no anaesthetic drops need to be used, and there is absolutely no contact with the eye at all, avoiding the spreading of infection or need for disposable instruments or scrupulous cleaning techniques. Perhaps surprisingly, however, many find the sudden puff of air more unpleasant than the gentle contact with the other devices, since the cornea is numbed with drops first anyway.

Taking a number of readings

It is usual to take a number of readings of pressure, and rarely is a diagnosis of glaucoma made on the basis of one alone. We know that the pressure within the eye varies from day to day, and indeed even throughout the course of the day, usually being at its highest on waking in the morning. If the examiner notes raised pressure on one occasion, in the absence of other abnormalities, he may well ask you to return for a pressure check on another day for a repeat check, possibly at a different time of the day.

Recently, observations have been made using experimental techniques of measuring the pressure in the eye directly, by means of inserting a small tube actually inside the eye. They suggest that the thickness of the cornea may have some effect on the pressure as measured by the techniques described above. Eyes in which the cornea is thin may have higher pressure than that measured, and for this reason sometimes the corneal thickness is also measured using ultrasound. This more specialist investigation is confined to hospital practice.

Defining normal pressure within the eye

The significance of raised pressure is very variable. Indeed, defining 'normal' pressure is itself something of a dilemma, since many eyes tolerate quite high pressures without damage, while others seem vulnerable to pressure that is usually regarded as being within the normal range. The average pressure in the eye is about 15mm of mercury (15mm Hg), but usually a pressure of 20mm Hg or below is regarded as being normal, in the absence of other signs of glaucoma. Interestingly, a difference in pressure between the two eyes is more significant than the absolute pressure in the eyes if they are both the same.

Measurement of pressure, then, is one of the mainstays of glaucoma diagnosis and management. Although it can be misleading when looked at in isolation, it still provides the major method of screening for glaucoma. In addition, it is the only one of the three parameters that can predict what might happen to the vision in the future, since assessments of the optic nerve and visual fields look at what has already happened.

George

George (age 67) attended his high street optometrist for a routine eye test after receiving a reminder from

18

the practice. He had been wearing reading glasses for several years, but otherwise had no eye problems. He realized when he got to the practice that he had actually not had a check for five years in spite of the reminders that had been sent to him. The optometrist found that his glasses did not need changing, but when he tested his pressure using the 'air puff' machine, which blew a short blast of air at the eye, it was slightly raised in each eye. He then asked to George to do a field test to check his peripheral vision, and this was normal, as was the optometrist's examination of the eye. George had no family history of glaucoma and was fit and healthy. The optometrist asked him to return the next week for a repeat test of the pressure. On this occasion it was completely normal. The optometrist reassured George that all was well, but reinforced the need to make sure he had his regular eye tests when contacted.

George illustrates a very common situation. Many people have single measurements of raised pressure, which may subsequently be normal when repeated. In the presence of a normal appearance of the nerve of the eye, and a full visual field, an isolated measurement of raised pressure is not in itself significant. It is important, however, in such a case, to be certain that it is just an isolated measurement, and the optometrist was careful to check the pressure again a little while later.

In George's case, the pressure was never very high, and indeed normal on repeat testing. Sometimes the pressure remains a little elevated, and in such cases the optometrist may choose to refer onwards to a hospital eye unit for further evaluation. George's case might be thought of as a 'false alarm', and this very common scenario should not provoke anxiety. More seriously, however, the history illustrates the possible dangers of not attending for regular eye checks when sent for. If George had turned out to have glaucoma, he could potentially have gone for five years without treatment through his failure to respond to appointments sent to him.

The appearance of the optic nerve

The appearance of the optic nerve as viewed by an examiner looking through the pupil with magnification is the second important parameter of glaucoma assessment. More specifically, it is the optic nerve head that is imaged, this being the point at which all the many nerve fibres that serve the retina are gathered together into the optic nerve, and leave the eye to pass backwards, eventually to the brain. The optic nerve in each eye contains approximately one million nerve fibres, and it is wonderful to think that, although they are obviously too small to see individually, this aggregation of the nerves, and the supporting tissues for them, can be viewed directly. Indeed, the eye is the only part of the body in which nerves and blood vessels can be directly viewed – perhaps this is why it is regarded as the 'window to the soul'! It is a useful analogy to think of viewing the optic nerve as being rather like looking at an electrical cable, which is made up of many thousands of component wires that are widely spread out, and come together to form a single trunk. It is the 'end-on' view of the trunk as it is formed that represents the optic nerve head.

As the many fine nerves join together to form the optic nerve, they acquire a coating, which speeds the conduction of impulses. This is rather like the bare wires of the electric cable acquiring a plastic covering as they form into the main trunk. In addition, there is supportive tissue around the fibres, and right through the centre of the optic nerve travel the main artery and vein that

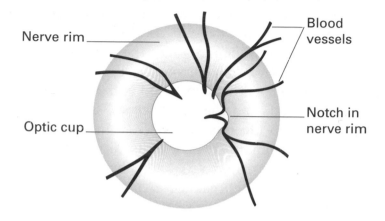

Figure 2 The optic nerve head

supply the inside of the eye. As the nerves lining the eye form into the main nerve trunk, they also turn backwards, since the main nerve then travels out of the back of the eye into the eye socket, and onwards to the brain. The appearance of the optic nerve head is shown in Figure 2. Looking at this illustration, it is apparent that within the end-on view of the nerve there is a central, concentric circular zone, and this is termed the *optic cup*.

Although not an infallible assessment of the nerve, an enlargement of this cup can represent damage to the optic nerve through glaucoma, and specialists often refer to the *cup:disc ratio*. This means the proportion of the whole optic nerve head (the 'disc') that is occupied by the 'cup' (the central circular zone). In a normal optic nerve, this is typically 0.2 to 0.4, while an enlarged ratio of 0.8 or 0.9 might be seen in glaucoma.

Unfortunately, nothing in life is ever as simple as this, and some people have a large cup:disc ratio without ever developing glaucoma. More significant in the assessment of the optic nerve head is whether the optic cup is symmetrically placed within the nerve, or whether there might be a notch in the cup, leading to a thin rim between the cup and the margin of the optic nerve head.

Another indicator of glaucoma is the presence of a tiny 'splinter'-shaped fleck of blood at the margin of the optic nerve head, and the presence of such a change strongly suggests the diagnosis. Once again, it alone cannot be relied upon, since it is usually transient and not present in the majority of those being tested.

It can be seen, then, that the assessment of the optic nerve head, though important in the diagnosis and monitoring of glaucoma, is not entirely straightforward, and open to some variation in interpretation between different observers. Add to this the fact that there are many different variants of the 'normal' optic nerve head appearance, together with a variation in appearance in the long- or short-sighted eye, and it is readily apparent that there can be some inaccuracies in diagnosis. Although the appearance of a nerve with advanced glaucoma may be quite obviously abnormal, and that of an entirely healthy nerve quite obviously normal, there are a large number of cases where the diagnosis may not be clear. Indeed, even so-called 'experts' in glaucoma may disagree about the health or otherwise of a particular nerve in some cases.

In an attempt to be as objective and accurate as possible in the assessment, various attempts to improve and automate analysis of the optic nerve have been made.

Using high powers of magnification, and different colours of light to illuminate the eye, it is possible to view the nerve fibres coating the inside of the eye directly. This can be done using the standard slit-lamp at which most eye examinations are made, and indeed this is an examination that is routinely undertaken by most specialists, should you be referred onwards for further examination. In addition, however, there is an ever increasing number of automated systems for analysing the optic nerve. Discussion of these highly sophisticated pieces of electronic technology is beyond the scope of this book, but basically they all are attempts to identify and record the appearance of the nerve in a reproducible manner, so that the accuracy of diagnosis can be improved, as well as the monitoring of any progression of the condition.

Some of these machines are based on photographic recording of the appearance of the optic nerve head, either using mono or stereo photography, while others use laser technology to scan the back of the eye and perform measurements of the thickness of the nerve fibre layer. They are all painless to have performed, and generally confined to hospital environments, mainly because of their huge expense and complexity. The science of optic nerve head imaging is currently rapidly evolving, and at the time of writing there is unfortunately no uniform technology that is used in all, or even most, units. In practice, at least the initial assessment of the nerve relies upon the clinical skills and experience of the examiner. In most cases, this will involve the use of either a hand-held instrument called an *ophthalmoscope*, or the use of an additional lens held in front of your eye, as you place your chin on the rest of the slit-lamp microscope.

Sarah

Sarah moved from the south coast to live nearer to her family. She had always been to her optometrist every two years for a routine check-up and had never been told she had any sort of eye problem. When she moved, however, her new optometrist examined her and felt that the appearance of the optic nerve was not normal. In spite of normal pressure in the eye and a normal field of vision, he felt that the abnormal appearance was sufficient to warrant further investigation, and referred Sarah to the local eye department. Here, after a number of further examinations and photographs, the eye specialist decided that the appearance of the nerve head, though somewhat unusual, did not represent glaucoma. He reassured her that there was no sign of glaucoma, but again emphasized the importance of regular checks.

Again, this sounds like a 'false alarm', and Sarah, having had no mention of glaucoma for many years, felt quite upset that the new optometrist had sent her off for a series of tests. Was he wrong in doing so, or should her previous optometrist have sent her many years ago? There is no easy answer to these questions, but the case illustrates a very common situation, where one practitioner may be quite happy with the appearance of the nerve (as was the hospital specialist after further investigation) while another might have concerns. The variability of what is normal is what causes the difficulty, and the first optometrist clearly felt that the nerve was healthy, and indeed its appearance had not changed over the many years he had been looking after Sarah. The new optometrist, however, without having seen her before, was less certain.

Not only does this illustrate how different practitioners may have different opinions, or thresholds for concern, but it also shows that often a diagnosis may need to be based on noticing a change in appearance, rather than simply on the appearance at one time. The purpose of the photographs taken at the hospital was to establish a baseline from which any possible future changes in appearance could be measured.

The assessment of the field of vision

The whole purpose of diagnosing and treating glaucoma is to maintain vision. The first sign of loss of vision is loss of some of the peripheral field of vision, and usually this is so slight at the time of diagnosis that the person with it is unaware of it. Indeed, it is the very gradual nature of the loss that makes it so difficult for someone to be aware of it, until it has become quite significant, since the tendency is for the eyes to adapt to the very gradual loss of field uncomplainingly. As the loss of field of vision begins to encroach on the more useful, central areas of vision, however, the reality becomes apparent, and it is impossible to put back what vision has been lost. Clearly, it is sensible then to prevent any such loss by diagnosing the condition before it gets to this stage or, even better, diagnosing it before any noticeable loss of field has occurred at all.

Modern techniques of measuring visual field are increasingly sensitive and sophisticated, and routine field tests to pick up early glaucoma are now widespread. In spite of this, it is estimated that up to 40 per cent of the important *ganglion cells*, which make up part of the optic nerve, must have been destroyed before even modern techniques can identify some loss of visual field. In other words, glaucoma is already well established before we can detect it. This is not as gloomy as it sounds, however, since if the condition cannot even be detected in its early stages, then it won't be causing symptoms. As long as it can be identified soon enough that treatment will prevent any noticeable visual loss, then no harm will be done.

The field of vision really is the gold standard by which diagnosis and treatment of glaucoma can be judged. It is all very well to ponder the niceties of the normal or abnormal optic nerve head appearance, or to speculate as to what 'normal' pressure in the eye should

25

be, but it is towards preservation of the field of vision that all efforts are directed. We shall see later how different individuals require varying levels of pressure control to achieve this, but ultimately it is the field of vision that determines the success or failure of management.

Let us consider, then, how this most important parameter of glaucoma assessment can be measured. In order to understand these measurements, we need to look first at what the situation is in the normal eye.

We all have a field of vision within which we can see. Although this may vary somewhat between individuals, it is obvious that none of us can see behind us without turning around, and that there are limits to the extent of how far to the sides and up and down that the eye can see. You can illustrate this by staring straight ahead, and concentrating on a distant object in the centre of your vision. If you then gradually move your outstretched arm from behind your shoulder in a large arc to move so that it is in front of you, while holding up your index finger, there will come a point at which you will first see the finger. For most people, this will be just after it moves in front of the shoulder, and this is a very crude assessment of the field of vision to the side of the eye.

If you try this again, but this time closing the eye *opposite* to the arm you are moving, you will find that the finger is still noticed at the same position. This is because the most peripheral perception of the finger will be by the eye on the same side as the arm that you are moving, and whether or not the other eye is open does not matter. If you then repeat the test again, this time closing the eye on the *same* side as the arm that you are moving, you will not see the finger until it is much nearer the centre of the body, since the opposite eye does not have a field of vision extending as far to the periphery on that side. This practical demonstration of visual fields shows us that the field of vision with both eyes open is much greater than that with only one eye open. This is because each eye, as well as covering a field of vision also perceived by the other eye, also serves an area that only it can see. Not only do we therefore have a larger field of vision with both eyes open, but we can only have proper depth perception through stereo vision in the area of the field that both eyes can see.

The practical implication of this in terms of glaucoma diagnosis is that it is important in testing the field of vision to measure one eye at a time. Otherwise, an area of missing vision in one eye might be compensated for by the other eye. Sadly, this is exactly the reason that some people present with advanced glaucoma in one eye: their fellow eye has often made up for the area of lost field, such that they are not aware of it.

What is it like having a visual field test?

Although a rough idea of the field of vision can be obtained in the manner described above, this is obviously not a very accurate or reproducible method of assessment. The earliest attempts to measure field were not very different to this, however, and the *Bjerrum screen*, which until about 20 years ago was still the routine for testing, was quite a crude assessment. It involved the examiner moving white targets on a black screen in from the side, until the observer became aware of them, and then marking on a paper the position that they were perceived. Not surprisingly, computers have taken over these days.

In a modern visual field assessment you will be asked to sit facing a bowl-shaped screen, with your chin on a rest, and looking forward at a central target. One eye is tested at a time, the other being covered over by a patch. Small circles of light are then projected on to the screen, one at a time, in different positions. You will then be asked to push a button each time a light is perceived. To improve the accuracy of the test, the computer is able to 'watch' that you keep looking straight ahead, rather than looking around to find the light. In addition, it will identify false results, such as pressing the button while there is no stimulus present. The machine can then print out a map of which lights you were able to see, and which ones you missed.

Beyond this, some machines are able to make even more sophisticated assessments of the vision. The one most frequently used within hospital eye departments is called the *Humphrey Field Analyser*, although many others exist. We know that the central area of vision is much more sensitive than the more peripheral areas. Again, you can demonstrate this to yourself quite simply: hold a small piece of type directly in front of one eye at a distance that you can read it, keeping the other eye closed. Then move the type sideways, while continuing to look straight ahead. You will notice once it has moved slightly away from the centre that you can still see the type, but are unable any longer to make out what it says. This is because the concentration of sensitive receptors in the retina is greatest where we need them most – the centre of vision. Some visual field analysers are able to allow for this, by projecting different sizes or intensity of lights to different areas of the visual field. It is even possible to identify the *threshold* of sensitivity of any particular part of the retina by repeatedly projecting lights until the dimmest or smallest that can be seen is identified. The computer can then print out this map of sensitivity, and even compare with a 'normal' field of vision or with previous fields undertaken by the same person on a previous occasion. This is an ideal way of monitoring any changes in the field of vision.

The testing of visual fields is a fascinating and evolving science. There are huge textbooks on the subject, and researchers whose whole lives are spent trying to refine the accuracy of such tests. The variation of testing strategies and machines is huge, and this can in itself cause confusion. For example, someone might have a field of vision test undertaken at his or her optometrist's that raises some concerns simply by not being entirely normal, but that when repeated using a different testing machine at the hospital, the field might seem completely acceptable. It is therefore very important not to be unduly concerned if you appear to 'fail' a field test, since this does not necessarily imply any disease.

Furthermore, many people find that their first attempt at a field test can give a poor result. Some machines do take some getting used to, and it is not unusual to find somebody's field of vision apparently improving, while in fact they are just becoming more familiar and comfortable with the testing procedure. If you wear glasses, it may be necessary for lenses to be put in the machine before testing to allow for this, since it is not possible to do the test while wearing glasses whose frames will reduce the field of vision. Not surprisingly, people with slow reaction times may find the test more difficult, as may others with arthritis of their hands, which makes it more difficult to press the button. Although an examiner will usually identify these difficulties, it is helpful to point them out if you have any concerns that he or she has not done so.

Do not worry about having a field test. It is not an exam, and there is no 'pass' or 'fail'! It is simply a way of comparing your field of vision with what is regarded as a normal average. Glaucoma is only one of many conditions that can affect the field, and many of these are quite innocent variations in our normal anatomy. For example, somebody with very prominent eyebrows, or perhaps rather heavy eyelids, might appear to have some of the top part of their field of vision missing, for quite innocent reasons.

Screening

We have seen the importance of early diagnosis, and how regular visits to the optometrist are important in this regard. Screening is simply a term used to describe the process of looking for a disease in a population without symptoms, rather than waiting for the disease to present. Clearly, there is no point in screening for a condition that presents with symptoms at the time of onset, an obvious example being acute appendicitis. In a condition such as glaucoma, however, where there are no symptoms until late in the disease, and that can be prevented from progressing if diagnosed early, it is very useful to undertake routine examinations of seemingly healthy people to try and make an early diagnosis. Indeed, it is the routine screening for glaucoma by optometrists that has seen the sharp decline in cases of severe visual loss from the disease.

Since the condition is one of increasing frequency with age, and is unusual below the age of 45, it is logical that such screening be commenced at around the fifth decade of life. It is at this age that many people begin to need reading glasses, and therefore many of them are in contact with an optometrist anyway. Ideally they should have an examination every two years to measure the pressure in the eye. With the increased availability of 'off the shelf' reading glasses at a variety of commercial outlets, however, many people are choosing glasses for themselves without the benefit of an optometrist's expertise. Although this in itself is not harmful, the failure to have a screen for glaucoma may well be.

DIAGNOSIS

Although screening is good advice for all those aged 40 or over, people who have a family history of glaucoma are certainly wise to have regular checks. Within the UK, eye tests are offered free to those who have close blood relatives with glaucoma, and to those who are at risk of glaucoma (such as those with ocular hypertension).

Putting all the information together

We have seen that the three main parameters of glaucoma diagnosis are measurement of the intraocular pressure, assessment of the appearance of the optic nerve, and analysis of the field of vision. In the majority of routine tests, these will all be normal, and the decision that there is no glaucoma is not difficult to make. The difficulties arise when one or more of these parameters is abnormal. We have already seen that any one of them can be different to what is regarded as normal, without this indicating anything wrong with the eye. Indeed, far more people with an abnormal field result do *not* have glaucoma than have the condition.

However, the whole purpose of undertaking such tests is to pick up early disease if it is present, and it is highly likely that your optometrist will suggest onward referral to an eye specialist within a hospital if he feels that any of the test results is suspicious enough on its own to warrant further investigation, or if there is a combination of factors that prompts concern. For example, a slightly raised pressure with a normal field of vision and healthy nerve appearance might in itself not be very worrying, but if the person's father had glaucoma, the slightly increased risk might prompt referral. Let us consider next what the outcome of such a referral might be.

4

Further investigations

If the diagnostic tests discussed in the previous chapter suggest the possibility of glaucoma, it is usual for any further investigation to take place within an eye clinic. Depending upon the local system, this may be arranged directly by the optometrist, or he may report to your own GP who would then initiate the referral.

What will happen at the eye clinic?

It may seem somewhat repetitive, but undoubtedly some of what has already been done by the optometrist will be checked again. This is not because of any doubts about the accuracy of the optometrist's findings, but because, as we have seen, making or refuting a diagnosis of glaucoma often involves looking at the variation in certain measurements. Consistently raised intraocular pressure, for example, is more significant than a one-off reading that is high, and similarly a visual field defect that is repeatable is more likely to be of significance than one that is not.

It is usual to begin assessment by taking a history of what has happened so far. Normally, since there are no symptoms, this is a collation of the optometrist's observations, but if you have recollection of the mention of raised pressure when you saw a previous optometrist, perhaps some years ago, then it is appropriate to mention this. In addition, you will be asked about any family history of glaucoma, and any general medical history that may be relevant. Some drugs can affect the pressure in the eye, and you should notify the clinic of any that you are taking. You may well be asked to provide a specimen of urine, to check for diabetes, and have your blood pressure checked.

The specialist examining you will, after measurement of your vision, make a close examination of the eye. In particular, as well as testing the pressure in the eye again, and observing the appearance of the optic nerve, he will also examine the eye for any particular features that make glaucoma more likely. For example, there are certain abnormalities of the drainage angle that predispose to raised pressure. Even though these may have been present since birth, they may not have any effect until some years later.

This examination will be undertaken at the slit-lamp, which is simply a sort of microscope used to view the eye in great detail. The person places his chin on a rest, and presses his forehead forward to touch a band, and this keeps the head steady while the examiner looks at the eye through a microscope with binocular eyepieces. The illumination is provided by a slit of light (hence the term 'slit-lamp'), which allows a better stereoscopic assessment of the interior of the eyeball. In assessing the drainage angle of the eye, he may use a special lens to inspect it, called a *gonioscope*. This lens is applied gently to the surface of the eye, after numbing drops have been put in so as not to cause any discomfort. The gonioscope consists of a lens within which is a small mirror, to allow the specialist to look at the reflected image of the drainage angle, rather as a toy periscope can be used to look around a corner. In so doing, he may see debris blocking it up, most commonly loose pigment that has detached from the back of the iris, or simply that the angle is rather narrow or poorly formed.

Although it is possible to view the optic nerve with a normal-sized pupil, the assessment is facilitated by enlarging the pupils using drops. This also allows inspection of the rest of the interior of the eye. Visual field defects can be caused by conditions other than glaucoma, and it is important to exclude such rare conditions as retinal detachment as causes of any loss of field of vision. When drops are used to dilate the pupils for such an examination, it is normal for the vision to remain blurred for some hours afterwards, and it is important to be aware that driving will not be possible until the effects have worn off.

Repeating the visual field

We saw in the previous chapter the difficulty in interpreting visual fields, particularly when the changes are borderline, and that there are a number of different machines available to do this. Many field analysers in high street optometrists' premises are designed to provide a rapid screening of the visual field that can be offered to everyone as part of the routine eye examination. They generally use a light of size and intensity that the eye would be expected to see, to plot whether there are any areas of field loss. We have seen, however, that it is also possible to analyse the field in even more detail, and assess the threshold of sensitivity of the retina in different places. This *threshold* testing takes longer, and requires more complex, expensive equipment. It is not the kind of test that would routinely be offered by an optometrist (although some do), and is generally reserved for the more detailed examination that is required in those people referred on to the hospital. Do not be surprised, therefore, if the field test is repeated, and seems somewhat more complex and time-consuming on this subsequent occasion.

Recording the optic nerve appearance

An important part of diagnosis and monitoring of glaucoma is the examination of the optic nerve head.

We have already seen, in the previous chapter, how this can be achieved. Although the precise practices vary between different units, it is normal to make some record of the nerve appearance, whether this be simply a diagram of what the examiner sees with the magnifying lens used at the slit-lamp, or one of the other forms of analysis using photography or laser measurements. In a condition that can be very slowly evolving, it is often useful to be able to look back at notes from many years ago, and compare the descriptions with the current assessments.

Often the organization of a clinic is such that you may have this assessment and that of the visual field undertaken first, perhaps by a specialist glaucoma nurse, before you see the eye specialist. Once again, the establishment of a baseline appearance of the nerve is a critical part of diagnosing and monitoring the condition. Although it may seem frustrating to be subjected to so many seemingly repetitive tests, it is time well invested for the future. Try to be a patient patient!

Other tests

The understanding of glaucoma, like most conditions, remains incomplete. We are now able to examine the eye in incredible detail, using technologies unavailable only a few years ago, but still the search continues for ever-increasing accuracy of diagnosis, and indeed simplicity of assessment from the person's perspective. From time to time, newer techniques are developed for just these purposes, some of which stand the test of time, while others become less useful as our knowledge evolves. For example, many years ago, it was common to admit people to hospital to monitor their pressure throughout the day, and sometimes in response to a large fluid input – the so-called 'water drinking test' – but this examination was subsequently largely discarded, proving to be of limited use. Only recently, elaborate assessments of the blood flow to the optic nerve were attempted, but again found not to be very useful in routine practice.

We saw in the previous chapter that recent work has shown that the thickness of the cornea may also be important in some people, if an accurate pressure measurement is to be achieved, and though not universal, such measurements are currently becoming more widespread.

It is clear, therefore, that there are changes in the investigations used to assess glaucoma, and the tests you may be asked to have undertaken will depend upon current thinking at the time you present. Some of these may be in the context of a research project, in which case you would, of course, be fully informed of this and have the choice of opting out if you wish. Although there is a temptation to deride some of the old-fashioned diagnostic tests, we should not forget that our current knowledge has evolved from them, and that many of our current practices will seem dated in due course. Overall, the trend in glaucoma diagnosis is for increased automation and machine-based assessments, but however much this trend develops, there is still the need for judgement as to how to analyse all the information that has been obtained. Do not regard yourself as a guinea-pig if offered tests other than those we have discussed, but appreciate that glaucoma is very much a condition about which our knowledge is still evolving.

Have I been diagnosed yet?

At the conclusion of all these tests, it is usually possible to decide one way or another whether glaucoma is present. If the diagnosis has been confirmed, your treatment will be discussed with you, and this is the subject of a later chapter. On the other hand, if the tests have shown that there is no sign of glaucoma, it is likely that you will be discharged, but you are still wise to continue your regular visits to your optometrist as before.

There still remains a minority of people, however, in whom the situation may not be clear, even after all the investigations. These people are often somewhat menacingly termed 'glaucoma suspects'! This term simply means that the specialist feels that there is no glaucoma at present, but that it would be wise to keep a watch on the person. Such a situation might arise if, for example, a small defect was detected on the field test, in the presence of normal pressure and nerve appearance. Although in itself the change would not indicate glaucoma, its progression over a period of time might do so, and for this reason the person would be recalled some time later to repeat the tests.

More common than the case of the 'glaucoma suspect' is the situation whereby raised pressure in the eye is confirmed, possibly on several occasions, but everything else appears normal. This is termed *ocular hypertension*, which is the subject of the next chapter.

5
Ocular hypertension

Ocular hypertension means high pressure in the eye, which is not glaucoma. The definition is clear, but in practice it can be difficult to distinguish from glaucoma. This is because, as we have already seen, the very early signs of glaucoma might be so subtle as to be difficult to identify, and it may be only if there is a change in the visual field or optic nerve head appearance that the diagnosis becomes apparent. There is no doubt that the levels of pressure that the eye can tolerate without damage vary in different people. Many eyes, for example, may have a pressure of 25mm Hg (remember that we regard normal as less than 20mm Hg) without ever developing glaucoma, and that this level of pressure is 'normal' for them. If a person presents with this pressure, then, and the visual field and nerve appearance are normal, it can be difficult to decide whether this is just their normal pressure, or whether they have not developed glaucoma *yet.*

The options therefore are either to treat the person anyway, or keep a watch for the earliest signs that glaucoma is developing, and then commence treatment. Although the former option seems attractive in some ways, it is worth bearing in mind that starting treatment usually commits the person to using drops in their eyes for the rest of his or her life, and to have continued monitoring. Although that is a small price to pay for preserving vision, it is not a decision to make lightly, if observation without treatment can still prevent any visual loss if changes are picked up early enough.

The approach to management of this situation varies between different clinicians, and indeed has changed with time. Twenty years ago, raised pressure was usually treated anyway, since the other diagnostic tests for glaucoma were not as sophisticated or sensitive as today. Since field defects had to be much more advanced before they could be identified, and testing was more prolonged, it was quite likely that extensive damage to the optic nerve might have occurred before diagnosis. With modern technology, we are able to monitor many of those with ocular hypertension who might previously have been diagnosed as having glaucoma, and realize that most of them will never develop the condition. This has in turn led to the strange paradox of some people who were diagnosed as having glaucoma many years ago being now told that in fact they just have ocular hypertension. Having been warned for years of the dire consequences of not using their drops, they are then asked to stop them! It is hardly surprising that many become confused, and sometimes a little annoyed, at this apparent contradiction.

Monitoring ocular hypertension

The usual strategy once ocular hypertension is diagnosed is to undertake regular monitoring. This normally includes checks of the intraocular pressure, together with an assessment of the optic nerve, and testing of the visual field. The frequency of review, and the personnel undertaking it, will vary from one unit to another, but usually annual review is all that is required. Should the pressure continue to rise, or any other new changes develop, then a decision may be made to commence treatment. Although the risk of somebody with ocular hypertension developing glaucoma is greater than that for somebody with normal pressure, when we consider the high incidence of glaucoma in the population as it ages, it is clear that anyway regular review is wise for everyone as they get older. The difference in ocular hypertension is that this is likely to be somewhat more frequent than the usual eye check every two years, and more likely to involve a more detailed and regular test of the visual field.

Certain factors may influence the frequency of review, and indeed lower the threshold for commencing treatment. For example, the presence of glaucoma in a close blood relative or identification of changes within the eye that can be associated with glaucoma may prompt the specialist to suggest treatment. The recognition that the intraocular pressure may actually be higher in those who have thin corneas than that measured by traditional methods may also influence the decision to treat.

The ocular hypertension treatment study

In an attempt to solve the perennial dilemma of which people with raised pressure to treat, and which ones to leave alone, a huge study – sponsored by the National Eye Institute in America – undertook a study in which over 1,600 people with raised pressure, but no other signs of glaucoma (i.e. with ocular hypertension), were monitored over a five-year period. Half of them were treated with drops to reduce their pressure by at least 20 per cent, while the other half had no treatment. The study showed that 4.4 per cent of those treated developed glaucoma, compared with 9.5 per cent of those who had no treatment.

Superficially, the case seemed to have been made for treating anybody with raised pressure, since only half as many of those treated developed glaucoma as those untreated. An alternative interpretation of the results, however, is that treatment did not prevent glaucoma in 4.4 per cent of those in the study, and that over 90 per cent of the 1,600 did not develop glaucoma anyway.

This then raises the question of whether all these people who would not have developed the condition anyway, should be exposed to the inconvenience, potential side-effects and complications, quite apart from the expense, of treatment. In some ways, the study raised as many questions as it answered, but certainly provided food for thought for both clinicians and those in the study.

Brian

Brian (aged 57) was found to have high pressure in his eyes at a routine examination by his optometrist. He had attended several times before, and on all previous visits the pressure had been normal. He was therefore surprised to hear that he had high pressure, and even more so to be referred onwards to the local hospital for further testing. After he had had the pressure measured again, and undertaken a field of vision test, a doctor examined him. This included putting drops in his eyes to dilate the pupils, and photographs were taken of the nerve at the back of his eye. The doctor concluded that, apart from the raised pressure, everything in the eye was normal. He suggested that it would be wise to repeat the measurements a year later, but that he needed no treatment.

Brian wondered what all the fuss had been about, since he had no symptoms, no other eye disease, and no family history of eye problems. He agreed, however, that it would be sensible to remain under review.

This is a fairly typical history of ocular hypertension. It is not surprising that Brian wondered why everybody was concerned, when he was completely free of symptoms. The majority of those with raised pressure never develop glaucoma, as was demonstrated by the study we described earlier. It is not possible, however, to be sure which people will develop glaucoma, and a raised pressure certainly increases the risk. The absence of symptoms is exactly the reason that such people require to be monitored, or the opportunity to treat early disease may be missed. Most units would suggest just an annual review of the pressure, field test, and nerve head appearance.

Khalid

Khalid was first told that he had high pressure in his eyes at the age of 54, and had been under annual review at the eye department of his local hospital ever since. At the age of 60, the doctor examining him told him that, although the pressure in his eyes had not changed, he now had glaucoma, on the basis of a change in the visual field test that he had done each time he visited. Khalid was still completely free of symptoms, but agreed to start treatment, which was a drop to be administered just once a day to both eyes. He continued this indefinitely, and so far there has been no further change in his field of vision.

This is again a common scenario. Initially a diagnosis of ocular hypertension was made, since the pressure in Khalid's eyes was raised, but the visual field was normal, as was the appearance of the optic nerve. A proportion of those with ocular hypertension subsequently develop glaucoma, and indeed detection of this is the entire purpose of follow-up. If changes develop such that glaucoma is diagnosed, this is often referred to as *conversion* to glaucoma, and treatment is then started. We know that glaucoma becomes more common with age anyway, and it may just be that ageing was the cause of Khalid's glaucoma, rather than the raised pressure alone. Perhaps it is best to think of ageing and raised pressure as both being risk factors for the development of glaucoma, as are a family history and certain specific ocular conditions mentioned earlier. Once diagnosed, it is almost certain that Khalid is likely to need his medication for life.

Very high pressure

Although there is no definition of what constitutes very high pressure, there does come a point at which few doctors would be happy to leave raised pressure untreated even if all other parameters for diagnosing glaucoma are negative. We know that the risk of developing glaucoma is proportionate to the level of pressure, but in addition it appears that when the pressure is more significantly raised, particularly when it is above 30mm Hg, that the risk of other events within the eye increases. These may include occurrences such as obstruction of the veins within the eye, leading to sudden reduction or loss of vision. Since such events have many other contributory factors, it is difficult to be certain of the significance of raised pressure as a causative factor, but in practice most doctors would recommend treating ocular hypertension when the pressure is greater than 30mm Hg regardless of the absence of other indicators.

Maria
Maria, aged 46, attended her high street optometrist for a routine eye check, and was found to have very high pressures in each eye (34mm Hg in the right, and 36mm Hg in the left). She had never had an eye test before, but had no problems with her vision, other than having just noticed some difficulty with close work, finding that she needed to hold papers further

away from her to see clearly. Her optometrist was concerned by the pressure, and arranged an early referral to the local eye department. Following further examination, and checking of her field of vision, the doctor told her that, apart from the raised pressure, her eyes were completely healthy. He explained that the difficulty in reading was nothing to do with the pressure, but simply a reflection of the normal loss of focusing ability that occurs with age. He advised Maria, however, that she should start to have drops to reduce the pressure in her eyes, since he felt that the pressure was so high that she was at risk if it was not lowered. She started drops once a day, which she continues to use. She has never developed glaucoma, even though it is ten years since the raised pressure was identified.

It would be easy to suggest that the treatment prevented Maria from developing glaucoma, but equally to imagine that she might never have developed it anyway. This is a question that could never be answered, since the clinical assessment was to start the drops, so we will never know if the disease would have developed without treatment. Often such dilemmas of management do present, and it is helpful for you, armed with the knowledge that you now have, to be involved in the decisions regarding treatment. Current practice would lead most doctors to advise treatment under these circumstances, but if the drops could not be tolerated, and more intervention would be needed to control pressure which might never be harmful anyway, the decision becomes more difficult. You should feel free to question your doctor as to why he feels treatment is indicated, and the potential risks involved either by leaving the condition untreated, or indeed proceeding with any particular treatment strategy.

Room for discussion

It will be very apparent from this book so far that the diagnosis of glaucoma is not always a certain one. The doubts about diagnosis, and dilemmas as to whether or not treatment is indicated, are highlighted in the situation of ocular hypertension. Translating risk assessments, cost/benefit ratios and global strategies for disease management into decisions for the individual concerned is always fraught. Most doctors are more than happy to discuss such questions with their patients on an individual basis, and certainly you should feel free to discuss the indications for treatment, particularly since it is likely to be for life. Equally, it is good practice to review the situation periodically, and consider whether in the light of any recent knowledge, and the clinical status of your own condition, changes should be made to the treatment plan. This could involve either commencing or stopping treatment, or perhaps seeking a different target of pressure reduction. In the next chapter, we shall consider exactly what treatments are available, and the possible benefits and problems with them.

6
Medical treatment of glaucoma

Treatment of glaucoma for the vast majority of people is medical. This means the use of drops, or occasionally tablets, rather than laser treatment or surgery. There is now a huge armoury of medications that can help in the control of the condition, and although there are still cases that require surgery, these are much less frequent since the advent of powerful medical remedies.

We discussed in the first chapter that there are different types of glaucoma, and how the condition of angle closure glaucoma is treated rather differently to the more common forms of glaucoma in which the pressure rise is more gradual and modest. The treatment of angle closure glaucoma, therefore, is covered separately in Chapter 8.

Strategies for treatment

The strategies for treatment of glaucoma are based on a variety of factors. The level of the pressure in the eye is obviously one but, in addition, the age and general health of the person, and extent of the condition, are also influential. Certain treatments may have specific side-effects that need to be avoided in particular individuals, precluding their use. For example, drops that come into the category of *beta-blockers* are likely to exacerbate any underlying breathing difficulties in those who have asthma. Some people may have other problems that stop them being able to apply eye drops at all, in which case other treatment methods may be appropriate.

The degree to which the intraocular pressure needs to be reduced is also variable. We have seen that some people lose visual field even when their pressure is within 'normal' limits, and obviously their pressure will need lowering below this to prevent further damage. Taking such factors into account, it is common practice to identify a 'target pressure' to which the pressure should ideally be lowered. Although this can be a helpful basis for treatment, the target may need to be adjusted if, for example, field loss is continuing in spite of the target having been achieved.

Increasing understanding of the condition suggests that reduction in the pressure of the eye may not necessarily be the whole aim of treatment, and some modern drugs try to increase the blood flow to the optic nerve. Increasingly, the concept of *neuroprotection*, which means simply protection of the optic nerve, is taking over from simple reduction in pressure.

Confusion over names

Before considering the drops used for treatment, it is worth trying to clarify the sometimes confusing way in which all drugs, whether they be drops, tablets, or anything else, are named. Broadly speaking, drugs can be divided up into different categories, based upon their mechanism of action, and their chemical structure. Within such categories, there is usually a variety of drugs, of roughly similar type, but differing somewhat in structure. This is rather like saying that there are a number of types of shampoo, all of which may do the same job, but may be marketed in, say, different fragrances. Within the category of beta-blocker drugs, for example, we find a host of different types, some quite similar to each other, and others that may have specific differences with which to distinguish them, such as not causing the breathing problems generally associated with this category of drugs.

47

Individual drugs of a specific and unique chemical composition are given a particular, unique name to describe them. This is called the *generic* name. As well as this name, however, the manufacturer will assign a brand name, just as the shampoo manufacturers will invent a more glamorous or descriptive name for their green shampoo with an apple fragrance.

This can all seem a little confusing, and is sometimes a source of concern to people, who find that the drop that they have been using for many years seems suddenly to have acquired a new name, whereas in fact the drug itself really remains unchanged. In addition, many of the brand names are chosen to maintain a corporate identity to the various products from one company, leading sometimes to somewhat unusual, and not necessarily easily memorable, names.

If in doubt, it is worth looking at the data sheet accompanying your bottle of drops, on which the drug will be described using its generic name.

How do the eye drops work?

Not all eye drops work in the same way, and we shall now consider the mechanisms by which they work. I shall return to the analogy we considered in Chapter 1, comparing the production and drainage of aqueous within the eye with the flow of water into a bath when the taps are turned on, and the plughole left open.

Currently, there are three main mechanisms of action of the drugs used in glaucoma.

The first is to reduce the pressure in the eye by reducing the production of aqueous fluid. This is the equivalent of turning the bath taps down, while the rate of water draining away remains the same, in which case we would expect the water level to go down.

The second method of reducing the pressure is to increase the outflow of fluid from the eye, either through the conventional pathway of drainage through the drainage angle, which we described previously, or through other pathways. We can think of this as unblocking the plughole in the bath, or even installing another one alongside it, to reduce the water level.

Finally, there is the third way of protecting the nerve, which is referred to as neuroprotection, and there are now a number of different drops that help to prevent the optic nerve from suffering cell death. Perhaps we could think of this as installing a tiled floor in the bathroom, such that any overflow of water would not cause harm anyway!

Some of the drugs we shall consider work in more than one way, and it is possible also to use combinations of them. Although the rapidly changing field of glaucoma treatment inevitably makes any study of individual drugs quickly become out of date, let us now consider some of the categories of drugs in more detail, bearing in mind these principles of how they may work.

Some technical details

Some of the following section may seem a bit technical for some readers. The intention is to give a little further information about specific drugs. You may prefer not to read all of this, and instead to study just the section on the drug you have been prescribed. Although the names are long, I have kept it simple!

Beta-blockers

These drugs may be familiar to anybody with high blood pressure, since they have been used for many years in tablet form for its treatment. Beta-blockers can also be used as eye drops, however, and they reduce the production of fluid within the eye. They usually need to be put into the eye twice a day, although there are some longer-acting varieties for which once-daily dosage is sufficient. They are extremely widely used in the treatment of glaucoma – and successfully so for many years. A whole host of different types exists, most of which have names ending in -olol – examples being *betaxolol, carteolol, levobunolol* and *timolol.*

These drugs are all generally well tolerated, and have certainly stood the test of time. They are, however, not usually suitable for those who have asthma, since they can exacerbate the condition, and can also slow the pulse unduly in susceptible individuals. Although the majority of people would not notice the effect, this can slightly limit exercise tolerance even in the healthy. A fit 78-year-old cyclist who was a patient of mine once complained that he got out of breath more easily when cycling up mountains since he had started taking beta-blocker drops! Because of their effects on the heart and lungs, these drops are usually avoided in those with heart failure or chronic lung disease.

A very rare side-effect of beta-blockers, but one that you might not attribute to eye drops unless specifically warned about it, is impotence. Although this common condition is very prevalent in the age group who may be taking drops for glaucoma, it is worth considering the drops as a possible cause of impotence, particularly if it develops at the time treatment is started.

Some of the adverse effects of beta-blockers can be avoided by the use of what are termed *cardioselective* drops. An example of these is betaxolol. Although they work in the same way as the other beta-blockers, they have less effect on breathing, but unfortunately also are sometimes rather less effective at treating the pressure. As so often in all treatments, it is often a case of balancing certain advantages against other disadvantages.

Alan

Alan developed glaucoma when he was 65, although otherwise was in good health. He had no history of chest disease and his specialist started him on timolol eye drops, which are a type of beta-blocker. He took these for several years without any problems, but at the age of 68 he began to get short of breath. After investigation by his own doctor, he was started on regular inhalers, which improved things dramatically. His doctor also asked him to stop using his eye drops, and consulted with the eye department looking after him to find an alternative treatment, which was successfully achieved. Alan was a little surprised that his eye drops might have been contributing to his chest problems, but was pleased with his improved ability to exercise without getting short of breath.

Asthma is often a condition of young children, which improves as they get older, but late-onset asthma is increasingly common too. Alan's doctor was right to stop his beta-blocker eye drops, since these can exacerbate asthma. They would not have been the cause of the asthma, since the changes they produce are reversible, but may well have been making things worse. Nowadays there are so many different types of eye drops that it is almost always possible to find an alternative. Even doctors do not always think that their patients may be using eye drops that are having effects on their general health, and it is therefore important when asked what medication you are taking to include your eye drops in the list.

Prostaglandin analogues

This is an unwieldy term for a group of drugs that has had a tremendous influence on glaucoma management in the last decade, and that now are generally used as the drug of choice in managing glaucoma. They work in a different manner altogether to the beta-blockers, and rather than reducing the production of fluid, they increase its outflow. They have the enormous advantage of needing to be instilled only once a day, and produce rapid and effective reduction of the pressure in the eye. We can think of these drugs as increasing the outflow from the bath by unblocking the plughole. To be more precise, how they actually work is by increasing the flow, not through the conventional drainage angle, but through drainage backwards in the eye eventually into the veins around it.

This clearly also gives the option of using them in conjunction with other drops, such as beta-blockers, if they are not sufficiently powerful on their own. Examples of this group of drugs are *bimatoprost, latanoprost* and *travoprost*. These are more familiarly known by their brand names of, respectively, Lumigan, Xalatan and Travatan. Note that while the beta-blockers tend to have names ending in -olol, the prostaglandin analogues have brand names ending in -an. The drug Xalacom consists of Xalatan combined with the beta-blocker timolol.

Other drugs that reduce aqueous production

We have seen that the group of drugs called beta-blockers can lower the pressure in the eye by reducing the amount of aqueous produced by the ciliary body. There are other drops that can do this. They do so, however, through a different biochemical process (the details of which we need not consider), such that their effect can be additive with those of the beta-blockers. This has the advantage that they can be used alone, or to supplement other drops, either when taken separately, or in a combined preparation.

MEDICAL TREATMENT OF GLAUCOMA

The drugs *dorzolamide* and *brinzolamide*, whose brand names are Trusopt and Azopt, are used either two or three times a day, depending on the pressure and which other drops they are used with. Generally, they are comfortable to take, with minimum side-effects. They are not quite as effective in most people as some of the other types of drops, and therefore are not usually the first choice for treating glaucoma, but can be very useful for those unable to take other types of drops, or as a supplement to these. The drug brand named Cosopt is a combination of timolol and dorzolamide.

Other drops that increase aqueous outflow

The earliest drug for treating glaucoma was *pilocarpine*, which works by increasing the outflow of aqueous from the eye. Although rarely used now in the treatment of the more common glaucomas, it is still the treatment of choice in angle closure glaucoma, which we shall consider in Chapter 8. The drug works by causing the pupil of the eye to constrict and, in so doing, pulls open the drainage angle to facilitate the outflow of fluid. Although extremely effective, it suffers from a number of disadvantages and side-effects. It needs to be administered four times a day, and can cause some aching over the eye and brow. Because the pupil is so small when pilocarpine is used, and unable to dilate when necessary, the vision in poor light is often affected, as is focusing. These effects are particularly troublesome in those who have cataracts. Once people have been taking pilocarpine for some time, the pupil remains permanently small, and this can make it difficult to examine the interior of the eye, or indeed to remove a cataract should this develop. For these reasons, pilocarpine has largely been discarded as a first choice for treatment of most glaucoma.

There are other drugs that increase aqueous outflow

without these side-effects, which fall into another complex-sounding group called *sympathomimetics*. Again, these are not generally used as first choice in glaucoma treatment on their own, but usually to supplement other treatment, or in people unable to tolerate other drops. Examples include *dipivefrine, apraclonidine*, and *brimonidine*. Some of these drugs may also have a direct neuroprotective action, as well as reducing the pressure in the eye. We shall consider what this means next.

Neuroprotective drops

We have briefly touched on the concept of neuroprotection already. It means simply what it says: protection of the optic nerve. This, of course, is what glaucoma treatment is all about, and reducing the pressure in the eye, which has until recently been regarded as the sole target of treatment, is now recognized as not being the whole issue.

The precise mechanisms of damage to the optic nerve in glaucoma still remain unclear, as we discussed in Chapter 1, and are probably variable between different individuals. However, recent research has identified certain drugs that may be able to protect the nerve by mechanisms apart from reducing the pressure. The detail of these mechanisms is complex, and still not fully understood, but development of such drugs probably offers the most encouraging prospects for improved glaucoma treatment in the future. The drugs that have recently been used to treat Parkinson's disease by protecting the parts of the brain involved in this condition can also be used to protect the optic nerve. In particular, the drug *memantine* would appear to offer neuroprotection, as do some of the sympathomimetic drugs we encountered earlier.

Side-effects of eye drops

It is fair to say that there is no drug in existence that is completely free of side-effects for all users, and eye drops are no exception to this. Some drugs have specific side-effects, to the extent that they are best avoided in certain susceptible individuals, and some of these are mentioned above. Although it is your doctor's responsibility to judge whether a particular drop is safe and suitable for you, you should inform him or her of any other medication that you are taking, and also report any side-effects that you notice, even if they are not those expected.

It is important to remember that drugs behave differently in different people, and the way that side-effects are recognized at all is by individuals reporting them. Do not therefore feel embarrassed to report seemingly unusual or minor symptoms, if these date from the start of your treatment. Even though it may not have been previously reported, other people may be suffering the same problem, and your specialist can then notify this to the appropriate agency, and hence provide useful information to other specialists and patients about the drug in question.

Some side-effects are less specific than, for example, causing shortness of breath in those with asthma, as is seen with the beta-blocker range of drops. In particular, the tendency to cause burning or stinging on instillation is common to many. Often this sort of sensation is very short-lived, and improves after a week or so of treatment, but if side-effects continue to the extent that you are not comfortable with the treatment, you should consult your specialist. Often it is just a case of switching from one brand of eye drops to a different one. Bearing in mind that treatment of glaucoma is usually for life, it is well worth experimenting with different treatments in order to find one that suits you.

Perhaps one of the more distressing side-effects that can occur from eye drops is the development of a type of dermatitis of the skin around the eyes. This can sometimes develop some months or even years after the drops have been used without a problem, though more commonly becomes apparent soon after the treatment is started. It presents with a redness, itching, and often quite severe swelling of the skin around the eye, usually extending slightly on to the cheek – in other words, in the precise distribution of where the drops might make contact with the skin, particularly if the eyes are rubbed. It is particularly striking if only one eye is being treated, since it is then isolated to that side, and the diagnosis is easy. Usually, however, both eyes are treated in glaucoma, and this might delay identifying the source of the problem. Often people are treated for conjunctivitis or other conditions before anybody realizes the culprit is the eye drops!

Treatment of this condition is the withdrawal of the offending brand of drops, and its replacement with another. On occasion, however, it is not the drug itself that promotes the reaction, but the preservative in the bottle of drops, which prevents them from decaying. Since the preservative (most commonly a drug called *benzalkonium chloride*) is the same in most drops, even a change in drops may not resolve the problem. If this is the case, it may be necessary to use drops without preservative, which means the use of single-use vials, rather than the more convenient bottle of drops. Alternatively, different treatment strategies may have to be considered, such as laser or surgery.

Elaine

Elaine was diagnosed by her optometrist as suffering glaucoma, and he quickly arranged for her assessment by the local eye department. They confirmed the diagnosis, and started her on a prostaglandin analogue drug, to be put in the eye once a day. Unfortunately, several days later she developed severe swelling around the eyes, with redness of the skin, and profuse watering. Worried that she had a severe infection, she attended the Accident and Emergency department, where, after advice from the eye specialist, a diagnosis of allergy to her eye drops was made. She was asked to stop all treatment, and reviewed in the eye department a week later. By this time, the swelling had settled, but the pressure in her eyes was raised still, since she was no longer having the eye drops. She was then started on a beta-blocker drop, but unfortunately the same thing happened again. Her specialist told her that he thought it was not the active ingredient of the drug to which she was allergic, but the preservative. He then started her on a different beta-blocker drop, to be taken twice a day from a *minim*. This is a small triangular-shaped plastic container, about 1.5cm long, with a removable cap. Each minim supplied enough drops to treat both eyes, after which she threw it away. She had to get her chemist to order in the minims specially for her, but established a routine of picking up a box of them once a month.

Poor Elaine had suffered a nasty allergic reaction not once, but twice. Allergy to preservatives is not common, but is highly likely in those who have had reactions to more than one drug, of different types. Although it is possible to test for the allergy by applying a test sample to the skin, this is not a routine practice unless the diagnosis is in doubt. The reactions suffered, though unpleasant, are not dangerous, nor do they lead to any permanent damage. The eye specialist felt it safe to leave Elaine with no treatment for a period of a few days while he was waiting to see if the swelling settled once the first drops had been stopped. Although obviously it is sensible not to delay treatment for longer than necessary, this strategy is quite safe. Indeed, had he not stopped all the drops, and instead switched her directly to the beta-blocker drops (which also caused a reaction), the diagnosis might have been confused. People are sometimes bemused by instructions that they must never stop their drops, to then find the specialist doing exactly this! The important thing is that he made sure she was seen again soon, to recheck the pressure.

How to put eye drops in

Although the diagnosis of glaucoma is not always an easy one to make, most people are more than willing to accept the importance of the regular use of drops if this decision is made. Many then worry about how to go about actually getting the drops into the eyes, and it is worth considering some practical tips concerning this.

The first consideration is when the drops should be used. Some need only to be inserted into the eye once a day, while others are required two, three, or – rarely – four times a day. Routine is the key to not forgetting, and although ideally the applications should be reasonably evenly spaced, this is not critical to the minute or even the hour. For example, a drop that needs to be inserted twice a day might be best put in after washing in the morning, and then again after cleaning your teeth at night. They may then be 14 or even more hours apart, but this is acceptable, and much preferable to trying (and failing) to space them precisely 12 hours apart, at times that are not convenient. I once had a patient who had to insert eye drops twice a day, and had been timing them so precisely that she took them two minutes earlier each day for the 30 days preceding the change to British Summer Time!

It is best, if at all possible, to put the drops in yourself. Many people worry initially that they might not manage this, but most are able to with a little perseverance and trial and error. To be reliant on somebody else for your drops to be inserted can lead to difficulties if that person is suddenly unavailable for whatever reason, quite apart from the inconvenience on a daily basis.

There are various ways of putting drops into the eye. For most people, the easiest way is to tip the head back slightly, pull down the lower lid with the finger of your left hand (assuming you are right-handed), and squeeze the bottle with the right hand to allow a drop into the little gutter that forms between the eyeball and the pulled-down lid. Do not try to score a 'bull's eye' direct hit to the middle of the eye, since not only is this not always possible, but it will be more uncomfortable if you do so. Some people prefer to put their drops in while watching in the mirror, and others actually lie down to put them in. Feel free to experiment!

It can be helpful, after instilling the eye drops, to press gently at the inner corner of the eyelids with your finger for about a minute, in order to prevent the drops from just draining away down the tear duct. This is not strictly necessary for most people, but is a good way of minimizing the amount of the drug that is absorbed into the body through the tear ducts in people who might suffer side-effects from them.

Various gadgets have been designed to help with putting drops in, and although most people will manage without, some find these helpful. They include small cradles for the bottles which have a mirror on them, so that you can view your eye directly as you squeeze the bottle. Other systems can help people with weak or awkward fingers, and it is worth asking your doctor or pharmacist if you are not able to manage with standard bottles.

If you have more than one type of drop to put in the eye, it is important not to wash the one out with the next one immediately after. Ideally, you should leave up to ten minutes between to allow absorption of the first type of eye drops.

It is inevitable that there will be some misses when you first start using drops, and you should not worry about this. It will do no harm to put the drop in again, if you are not sure whether any went in. Storing the drops in the fridge to keep them cold can help you tell whether the drop went in properly, although some people find cold drops a little more uncomfortable. It is important anyway to pay attention to their storage, and follow any instructions in the accompanying data sheet carefully. Although most drops do not have to be kept refrigerated, you should not allow them to be exposed to excessive sunlight and extremes of temperature. Do not forget to take them on holiday!

Most people realize the importance of using the drops regularly and comply well with their treatment. If, however, you do forget occasionally, do not panic. Missing one drop from time to time is unlikely to have any serious effect, but the effect can be cumulative if this becomes a regular occurrence. If you realize a few hours later that you missed a drop (or cannot remember if you did), it is perfectly reasonable to put in another drop. Do not miss out on your drops on the day you go for a check-up, since it is then impossible to know whether the drops are working or not.

7
Laser and surgical treatment

By far the majority of those with glaucoma are treated using drops, but there are times when either laser or surgical intervention is appropriate. Although generally this is when drug treatment alone is either unsuccessful or insufficient, there are specific types of glaucoma best treated using these techniques. Some people think of any operative procedure as being a 'last resort', while others regard laser or surgery as simply an alternative to the inconvenience of daily drops. Although surgery may sometimes be necessary because everything else has failed, and although it may also be a way of stopping drops, it is better to think of the medical and surgical treatments as being complementary. They both have pros and cons, and we shall consider these in this chapter.

Laser treatment

Ever since Goldfinger tried to kill James Bond by cutting him in half with a laser beam, the world has been fascinated by laser. Many people are enthusiastic to have any treatment associated with the technology, and it certainly does have a place in the management of glaucoma. Perhaps the most effective use of the laser is in the treatment of the rare form of glaucoma called angle closure glaucoma, which we have mentioned earlier, and laser treatment of this condition is discussed in Chapter 8.

Laser is also used in the treatment of the more common open angle glaucoma (POAG), although it is usually treated with drops. The procedure that is used is called a *trabeculoplasty*, and this simply means changing the shape (*-plasty*) of the trabecular meshwork. The meshwork is the area within the drainage angle through which the aqueous normally drains. By directing laser spots just in front of this drainage meshwork, a small amount of scarring can be created in a very controlled manner, so as to pull open the meshwork that is not draining fully. The type of laser used for the procedure is usually an *Argon* laser, and the procedure is therefore often referred to as an *Argon Laser Trabeculoplasty* (ALT).

In practice, this is not an unpleasant procedure to have done. The person sits at a machine very similar to the standard slit-lamp examination microscope, and drops are put into the eye to make it numb. A small contact lens is then held on the eye by the surgeon, coupled to the eye through some sticky, clear fluid. The lens contains a small mirror within it, to allow the surgeon to direct small spots of laser to the correct place. During treatment, the person is aware of sudden very bright flashes of light as approximately 50 individual pulses of laser are delivered. The whole process takes 10 to 15 minutes, after which the person being treated is usually asked to wait for a little while to recheck the pressure. They will be given anti-inflammatory drops to take for a week or so after.

The procedure is quick, almost painless, and usually effective. Sometimes one application of laser is not sufficient, and a second treatment is applied a month or two later. Unfortunately, the technique is not suitable for all individuals. In some it is simply not possible to access the area of meshwork adequately to apply the laser, while in others the laser does not cause sufficient reaction to have any effect. There are specific subtypes of glaucoma in which this form of laser is most likely to be successful, but again this is not always entirely predictable. The main drawback to laser treatment of glaucoma is its lack of permanent effect. Many of those who initially have a good response later develop a recurrent rise in pressure. Although the laser treatment can be repeated, it will not always continue to control the pressure in the long term.

As a supplement to medical treatment, laser can be very useful. In particular, those people who may already be having treatment with two types of drops, and still have slightly high pressure, may achieve good control following laser treatment. It can also be useful, however, for those who simply cannot take drops, for whatever reason. This may include those with bad arthritis who are not able to handle the bottle, those who are allergic to all the various preparations of drops, or even those who cannot reliably remember to use their eye drops. This latter category may include those with a frenetic lifestyle and those with dementia.

Although in certain cases laser may well be a choice over treatment with drops that proves to be more convenient, it is important to stress that it is still a surgical procedure, and therefore carries some small risks, as well as the possibility that the effect will not be sufficient, or will be short-lived. Although complications from the laser are rare, it is possible to suffer temporary raised pressure afterwards, and even to potentially damage the angle in the process. Like any other treatment, it is important to weigh up the risks and benefits in your particular case, with the surgeon undertaking the laser, before proceeding.

Drainage surgery (trabeculectomy)

The concept of drainage surgery may seem to be taking the analogy of the bath just a little too far, but this is exactly the term that is used for a group of operations

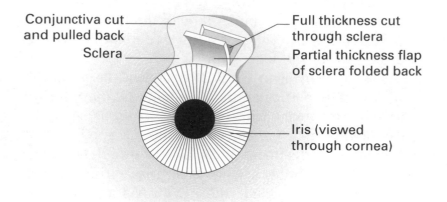

Conjunctiva cut and pulled back
Sclera
Full thickness cut through sclera
Partial thickness flap of sclera folded back
Iris (viewed through cornea)

Figure 3 Drainage surgery

that can be undertaken to lower the pressure in the eye. The term refers to the process of creating an alternative pathway from the eye, through which the aqueous may flow. In the bath analogy, this would be the equivalent of installing a new plughole in the bath – perhaps this is the point at which the analogy *is* stretched too far!

The traditional way that this is undertaken is to split a small, rectangular-shaped segment of the sclera of the eye, which is the white coating of the eyeball lying underneath the conjunctiva, into an inner and outer layer. Only three sides of the rectangle are cut, so forming a thin flap from the outer layer of the sclera, which can be folded back, hinged at the uncut edge, as shown in Figure 3 (above).

Underneath the flap, a small cut is then made through the remaining, deeper part of the sclera, so as to actually enter the eye, whereupon the aqueous fluid gushes out through it. A small hole is also cut in the iris underneath, in order to prevent it just blocking up the new drainage channel. The outer hinged flap is then placed back in position, to lie over the inner, perforated part of the sclera, and it is sutured back in place. The conjunctiva, which requires to be cut and pulled back to facilitate the dissection, is also stitched back. This then leaves a new pathway of drainage for the aqueous fluid: as well as draining through the normal drainage angle, it is also able to pass through the perforation in the inner part of the sclera and then leak around the edges of the flap in the outer leaf of the sclera, to collect underneath the conjunctiva. The whole procedure is undertaken underneath the upper lid and, on lifting the lid, a small blister is often seen, which represents the collection of fluid underneath the conjunctiva. From here, the fluid can drain away via the blood vessels in the conjunctiva.

Although this might sound complicated, it is really just a way of creating a controlled leak of fluid from the eye. The name given to this whole operation is trabeculectomy, and for years this has been the mainstay of glaucoma surgery. It is less commonly performed now than ten years ago, since the development of powerful drops to control glaucoma has allowed many people to be treated with drugs. It remains, however, a useful technique, and some recent refinements to the operation have made it even safer and more effective than when it was first introduced.

Antimetabolites

One of the main drawbacks to the trabeculectomy operation described above is that it is possible for the new drainage channel created to close over. Indeed, it may seem surprising that it does not always do so, if we think that normally tissues that have been cut will heal themselves. The reason that the flap of sclera does not usually heal over is that there is a flow of aqueous fluid around it (and indeed actually through it since it is so thin). In addition, the blood supply is poor compared with other tissues, which also impairs healing. Think how long a graze or cut to the shin, where the blood supply is poor, takes to heal compared to one on the arm or leg.

Whereas a surgeon will normally want wounds to heal following an operation, it is this very wound healing that can compromise the effect of the trabeculectomy operation, and in particular the development of scar tissue underneath the conjunctiva, which may seal off the free drainage of aqueous. This problem is particularly common and troublesome in races who have a tendency to produce excessive healing tissue, and most especially in Afro-Caribbeans. Those who have already had either previous surgery or injury to the eye are also more likely to develop such scar tissue, as are those who have had prolonged exposure to some eye drops. The effect of such healing over of the new drainage channel is that the pressure rises again: the operation then fails to achieve its objective. Such failure can occur as early as a few weeks after the operation, or may happen months or even years later.

Various attempts have been made to modify this healing, and prevent such failures. Sometimes this can involve some further minor surgical adjustment of the operation, usually a few weeks later. If, for example, the surgeon notes that there may be developing sufficient scar tissue to risk sealing off the little blister underneath the conjunctiva, into which the aqueous drains, he may gently free up this tissue, using a small needle. This can be done in the outpatient setting, using the slit-lamp. The procedure is known simply as *needling*.

More proactively, however, drugs are available that can be applied to the eye at the time of the operation, and in the first few weeks after, which prevent scarring developing in the first place. These are referred to as *antimetabolites*. They inhibit normal healing, by interfering with the normal replication of cells. They can also be used in the treatment of cancer, when they act in the same way by preventing growth of the cancer cells. There are different ways of using these drugs in glaucoma surgery. Either they can be applied to the tissues around the operating site at the time of the operation, or they can be injected afterwards. Some surgeons only use them during the operation, while others reserve them for use later, particularly if there are signs that the new channel may be blocking up. The two most commonly used are called *5-Fluorouracil* and *Mitomycin-C*.

The use of antimetabolites has certainly improved the outcome from glaucoma surgery, particularly in difficult cases, but there are specific risks with them, which is why they are not used in all instances. The delicate balance between wound healing being sufficient to allow the operation to heal, but not excessive such that the drainage channel closes off, is the problem. While scarring under the conjunctiva is a bad thing, and likely to lead to failure of the operation, *some* healing is essential, to allow the conjunctiva to heal back into its natural position. If too much antimetabolite is used, then not only may the conjunctiva fail to heal, but it may become so thin and fragile that it can tear or allow infection into the eye. The cornea is adjacent to the operation site, and damage to the outer surface of it can occur from the drugs. Thankfully, modern surgery draws on the experience of the early use of these drugs, and the doses and techniques of application are now accurately controlled so as to minimize such risks.

Variations on a theme

There are some risks associated with glaucoma surgery, and these are discussed in some detail below. In an attempt to minimize in particular those associated with excessive drainage of fluid from the eye, variations on the theme of drainage surgery have developed. In particular, the concept of *non-penetrating glaucoma surgery* has evolved. The principle behind this is that a procedure similar to a trabeculectomy is undertaken, but instead of entering the eye by removing a full thickness segment of the sclera, some of the deeper tissues are left intact so that there is no true penetration into the interior of the eye. Instead, the drainage occurs through the very thin remaining sclera. Technically, this is more challenging surgery, and usually takes longer to perform. Some surgeons favour it over the more conventional trabeculectomy operation, while others are more sceptical about its advantages. Although the names seem complex, it is worth mentioning that there are variants of non-penetrating glaucoma surgery termed *deep sclerectomy* and *viscocanalostomy*, which may be referred to if your surgeon feels these are appropriate for you.

What is it like having a glaucoma operation?

Let us now consider the experience of having a glaucoma operation. Usually this is undertaken under local anaesthesia, without the need to go to sleep, although some people prefer a general anaesthetic if they are particularly anxious.

Although there are variations in the technique of giving a local anaesthetic, the principle is the same for all. First, a drop is put in the eye to numb it, following which some local anaesthetic is injected around the tissues of the eye. This can be done either with a conventional needle, or using a blunt, curved pipe which is used to inject through a small nick which is made in the conjunctiva. Whichever technique is used, it is not particularly uncomfortable, although obviously a little sharp for a few moments. The anaesthetic not only numbs the eye, but paralyses the muscles that move it, so making the procedure easier for the surgeon. Operating on a moving target can be difficult!

Once the anaesthetic has had a few minutes to work, the operation commences. Do not be surprised that there is still usually some vision present until the surgeon switches the bright light of the operating microscope on. Once this occurs, you will not see anything of the surgery.

During the operation, the eyelids are held gently open by a small clip, so that you do not have to worry about blinking. It is perfectly acceptable even to gently close the eyes while the surgery is going on. Although it may feel closed because the anaesthetic is acting, the eye being operated on will actually remain open because of the clip. Try to avoid squeezing the eyes, however, since this can be more uncomfortable, and also more difficult for the surgeon. In order to keep the area of the operation sterile, a clean drape is placed over the face, and only the eye being operated on will be exposed through a small hole in the drape. It is lifted off your mouth, however, and usually extra air is piped under the drape to prevent any feeling of claustrophobia.

A glaucoma operation takes around 15 to 20 minutes, but may take longer if enhancements such as the use of the antimetabolite drugs discussed above are used. During this time, you will need to lie back on a couch, and keep fairly still. This does not mean being rigidly immobile, and nor is it necessary to lie back absolutely flat. If, however, you find it difficult to lie back, or you have a bad tremor for whatever reason, it is helpful to draw this to the attention of the surgeon before the operation. You may be someone who is better off having a general anaesthetic for the operation.

At the end of the procedure, a protective shield is placed over the eye, to prevent accidental injury for a few hours afterwards. If local anaesthetic has been used, it is usual for there to be some double vision as it wears off. This is because it takes a while for the muscles that move the eye to recover, and so the two eyes will point in different directions until such recovery is complete. Do not be worried about this, nor by the fact that the vision in the operated eye will be blurred.

It is normal for vision to remain reduced in the eye for some days or weeks afterwards, for a variety of reasons. First, the drops that are used before and after the operation paralyse the normal focusing muscles within the eye, and also widen the pupil such that it does not react to light. In particular, this can lead to dazzle and glare, and difficulty in bright lights, when normally the pupil would constrict to compensate. In addition, however, the operation does change the shape of the eyeball, particularly in the early post-operative period. This is because the drainage of fluid from the eye leaves it less inflated, and as a consequence the depth of the chamber between the cornea and the lens is often reduced initially. This affects the optics of the eye to make it somewhat more short-sighted than it was, at least until the situation has stabilized. This may take from a few days up to several weeks. Do not be tempted to go and buy new glasses at this time, since although they may improve the situation for a while, they will need changing again later if prescribed before the situation is stable.

Side-effects and complications

There is no surgical procedure without some risk of complications, and glaucoma surgery can lead to problems. Before we consider some of the things that can go wrong, let us first consider some of the usual side-effects that often accompany the surgery.

We have considered already the temporary blurring of vision that accompanies glaucoma surgery, and that this can take some weeks to resolve. Often, though, some change in the refraction, however slight, may be permanent, as the eye adopts a new shape. In this case, it may be necessary to have a change of glasses, or even to start wearing glasses when they were not needed previously. This latter scenario is relatively unusual.

Another frequent side-effect of glaucoma surgery which, though rarely serious, can be troublesome to some people, is the sensation created by the formation of the 'blister' of conjunctiva underneath the upper lid, into which the aqueous now drains. Many people notice a sensation of grittiness, as if something is stuck underneath the eyelid as a result of this. It is particularly noticeable in the first few weeks after the surgery, when sutures that are used may irritate the eye. Modern sutures are so fine that they usually cause little irritation, but certainly it is not uncommon for some sensation to be present. In those whose eyes are very sensitive or suffer from poor tear production, this can be uncomfortable.

The blister of conjunctiva is intentionally created underneath the upper lid, where it causes least discomfort, and is least noticeable. On occasion, it can extend further and become visible when the lids are open. From an appearance point of view, this is rarely sufficient to be of concern, but some people worry at its development if not forewarned of the possibility.

True complications from glaucoma surgery are relatively rare, and the majority are the result of either excessive or inadequate drainage from the newly created system. Particularly in the first few days after surgery, it is possible for too much aqueous fluid to drain from the

71

eye, in which case the front chamber of the eye between the cornea and the iris can become shallow, or even flat. The reason for this is usually excessive leakage, usually from the wound in the conjunctiva, before it has had a chance to heal. Sometimes this may require attention, either applying a contact lens to the eye to put pressure on it, or even inserting an extra suture if the leak is marked.

The consequence of excessive drainage from the patient's perspective is that the vision remains very blurred, and there may even be a sensation of leakage of fluid from the eye. This is not a cause for panic, and the problem can usually be quite easily managed. If the pressure remains low for a while, then it is possible for the inner lining of the eye at the back to separate from the outer coating. This leads to further disruption of the vision, but thankfully it normally reattaches itself as the pressure builds up again.

Inadequate drainage from the eye is usually manifest by gradually increasing pressure over the weeks following surgery, to the point when it is necessary to use glaucoma drops again to control it. This does not necessarily imply failure of the procedure, and indeed it is often the case that surgery is undertaken to supplement the effect of drops, the expectation being that after the operation the pressure will be controlled through a combination of the surgery and resumed medical treatment. Sometimes, however, the pressure rises as excessive healing takes place, in the manner we described above, and this can necessitate intervention, such as the needling we discussed, or intensive application of steroid drops to minimize the scarring.

A routine part of a glaucoma procedure is to cut a small window in the iris adjacent to the site of drainage, in order to prevent the iris simply plugging the new drainage channel. The iris has a very good blood supply, and it is not surprising, therefore, that bleeding can occur following this. Although precautions are taken to minimize the chances of this, it is possible for enough blood to form in the eye that the vision is affected, particularly in those taking blood-thinning agents. The average volume of the small chamber at the front of the eye is 0.25ml, and it is not difficult to appreciate that only a minimal volume of blood can occupy this. If such bleeding does occur, it can usually be left to settle spontaneously, although this takes some days.

Other complications from glaucoma surgery are even less common. Infection is always of concern in any post-operative situation. Just as the surgeon and others involved in your care will do all they can to minimize the risks of infection, you too can play your part. Avoid contamination of the eye during the first few weeks after an operation by ensuring that you wash your hands carefully before instilling the routine post-operative drops, and avoid rubbing the eye. Although you do not need to isolate yourself at home, do try to avoid obviously dirty environments.

If an infection does develop in the early stages after surgery, it is important that you seek early attention. In the extremely rare condition of *endophthalmitis*, an infection actually penetrates to the inside of the eye, and this requires urgent treatment in order to prevent loss of vision. It is heralded by onset of pain, rapid worsening of the vision, and usually significant swelling of the eyelids.

Even when the eye has fully healed, it is important to be aware that the thin blister of conjunctiva is potentially a portal of entry for germs into the eye. Particularly if it is very thin, as may be the case if antimetabolites were used, a simple conjunctivitis may turn into something more serious if it is not promptly dealt with. Do not become over-anxious about your eye after surgery, but be alert to changes in comfort or vision.

Finally, there is a significant risk of cataract developing, or being accelerated by glaucoma surgery. This leads to a reduction in vision, which can be treated by cataract surgery, in which the cloudy lens of the eye is exchanged for a new, clear, artificial lens. The results are generally excellent. Since cataract is so common, particularly in the ageing population, it is often difficult to know how much the glaucoma surgery has contributed, since the two conditions often coexist. Indeed, if cataract surgery is planned anyway, it is possible to combine it with a trabeculectomy operation.

Elaine

As we saw (page 57), having suffered initial allergic reactions to drops, Elaine started preservative-free drops, using disposable minims, and had no further problems with discomfort or swelling of the eyelids. Her pressure was well controlled, and the visual fields remained completely unchanged for several years, as did the optic nerve appearance. After about four years on treatment, however, her specialist noted a slight increase in the pressure in her left eye, and arranged for her to have an earlier review than usual. The pressure continued to rise, however, and when she next had a visual field test undertaken, there was a very small change, which the specialist felt was due to progression of the glaucoma. She had noticed no change at all in her vision, but after discussion about the likely further loss of vision if this situation was left uncontrolled, she agreed to have surgery. This was performed under local anaesthetic as a day-case. Elaine found the whole process surprisingly easy and comfortable, but was disappointed the next day to find her vision very blurred in the eye, even though she had been warned of this. Her glasses made no improvement, and for approximately eight weeks the vision remained misty. At the end of this time, her specialist told her that she could have her glasses changed, and following this her vision was as good as before the surgery (but no better!), and she no longer needed any drops to control the pressure. The specialist told her that the pressure in the eye was now perfect at 14mm Hg.

This is a very typical case of initial control of the condition with drops, which subsequently requires surgery. In Elaine's case, her inability to tolerate any drops with preservative in them restricted the medical options open to her, but surgery is usually required whatever the reason for failure of drops. Trabeculectomy is not an operation from which patients usually note any benefit, other than sometimes being able to stop their drops, since its purpose is to arrest progress of the condition, rather than reverse change that has happened. This is indeed the very nature of all glaucoma treatment, but it is important to stress that surgery will make the vision worse, at least for a while. Even forewarned of this, people are often surprised by it, particularly if comparing notes with those who have had cataract surgery, who generally notice an almost immediate improvement. It is often only when the glasses are changed that the vision recovers properly, and this should not be done too soon while the situation is still changing. Once again, we see the need for patience.

Valves, tubes and other implants

A different approach to surgical lowering of pressure in the eye is the insertion of a small, plastic tube into the front of the eye, which is used to drain the aqueous to an external area underneath the conjunctiva. A variety of devices exists, some of which contain a valve, so that drainage only occurs once the pressure in the eye is above a certain level, while others are simply narrow tubes, connected to a sort of plate, under which the fluid can collect. The advantage of the valved system is that there are less problems of excessive drainage of fluid, such that the front chamber of the eye becomes shallow, or even flat. On the other hand, the simpler tubes usually achieve lower pressures.

The concept is simple, but the surgery is challenging. It is undertaken by a relatively small number of expert glaucoma surgeons, and usually reserved for cases in which conventional surgery has failed. The risks with the procedure are similar in nature to those of trabeculectomy, but in addition there are the dangers of the tube either damaging the fragile inner lining of the cornea, or even extruding from the eye. Although precautions are taken to avoid it, the risks and consequences of excessive drainage of fluid in the early post-operative period do appear to be increased over routine trabeculectomy surgery. In cases of trabeculectomy failure, however, or in eyes prone to recurrent inflammation or those in whom the drainage angle is blocked by abnormal blood vessels, the insertion of a tube may offer the best chance of success.

Ciliary body destruction

Some cases of glaucoma are particularly difficult to treat, and even the medical and surgical procedures described above fail to adequately control pressure. Under these extreme circumstances, it may be necessary to actually damage or destroy the part of the eye responsible for producing aqueous, which is called, as mentioned earlier, the ciliary body. This is quite a radical step to take, not only because the damage is permanent, but also because it is not possible to accurately judge how complete the destruction is. If all aqueous production ceases, then the eye will go soft, and may shrink to a somewhat unsightly degree. Inadequate treatment, of course, will not have the desired effect. Though not exclusively, the technique is therefore mainly used in eyes that have become blind or nearly so, in an attempt to reduce very high pressure that is causing pain.

The destruction can be undertaken using either a freezing probe, applied to the eye a few millimetres behind the edge of the cornea, or using a laser. The freezing technique is called *cyclocryotherapy*, while the usual laser technique is *cyclodiode therapy*. Both are undertaken using a local anaesthetic to freeze the eye. There is often some discomfort after the procedure, although it is painless at the time. It is possible to have some control over the amount of ciliary body that is destroyed, simply by varying the area over which it is applied. It is normal to err on the side of destroying too little, and therefore apply a number of treatments until the pressure is controlled, rather than risk complete shutdown by treating it all at once. Unfortunately, the long-term effects are not immediately apparent, and sometimes further treatment is required a while later if some recovery of the ciliary body occurs, while in others the pressure may continue to fall even years after treatment.

Treatment of childhood glaucoma

Although the medical treatments discussed in the previous chapter can be used in children, as in adults, the treatment of childhood glaucoma, and in particular that of congenital glaucoma, usually involves surgical intervention.

We saw earlier that the signs and symptoms of glaucoma in babies include enlargement of the cornea, profuse watering and sensitivity to light, reduced vision, and sometimes the wandering of the eyes known as nystagmus. If the diagnosis is suspected, then an examination with the child asleep under a general anaesthetic is needed, in order to examine the eye more completely, and assess the pressure within it and the appearance of the optic nerve. Babies and young children can obviously not co-operate with all these assessments while still awake. If the diagnosis is confirmed, the surgeon will usually undertake further surgery at the time to try and increase the drainage of fluid from the eye. The examination, and possibly the treatment also, are likely to need repeating, and the disease needs close monitoring, as does the visual development of the child.

A number of surgical options are available, which depend upon the severity of the condition, and the underlying cause. These include all of the procedures we have described already for adults, but in addition other treatments exist that are only used in children. These include *goniotomy*, whereby a special blade is used to cut open the drainage angle that has not developed properly, and *trabeculotomy*, which is a way of creating an alternative drainage pathway, similar to trabeculectomy, but not actually involving cutting out any tissue.

Management of childhood glaucoma is a highly specialized field. The condition is relatively uncommon, and there are therefore only a few sufficiently experienced to deal with it. It is quite likely, therefore, that if your eye unit does not have a doctor who treats childhood glaucoma, your child will be referred to somewhere that does. Some of the monitoring in between visits to the childhood glaucoma specialist may take place at the local eye unit and, as your child grows

78

up, management is likely to be handed back to them, in order to minimize as much as possible travel to hospitals further away.

There is sometimes an underlying abnormality of the eye responsible for glaucoma in childhood, which on rare occasions is associated with other conditions affecting parts of the body other than the eye. In addition, the possibility of the condition being hereditary is much greater than in other more common forms of glaucoma, and for these reasons access to a geneticist is helpful. Once again, these facilities may only be available in centres that specialize in childhood glaucoma.

There are many surgical options for management of glaucoma. Even those described above do not comprise the full spectrum of variations available, and individual surgeons may have particular preferences for one technique over another. The common goal of all of them is to lower the pressure in the eye, and disturb the vision as little as possible in the process. There is no doubt that glaucoma surgery is less common these days than even ten years ago, but it offers a very effective treatment, and you should not be perturbed if this becomes the best treatment option for you.

8
Angle closure glaucoma

In this chapter we shall consider angle closure glaucoma. This is so different to the other types of glaucoma, both in its presentation and treatment, that it is really best regarded as a completely different condition. Although it shares the common pathway of nerve damage through raised pressure, this is more or less where the similarities between it and the other glaucomas end. Although the presentation is more dramatic, the condition is usually quickly curable, without the need for lifelong treatment with drops and indefinite follow-up. I often think of it as the eye equivalent of acute appendicitis – once treated, never to return!

What is angle closure glaucoma?

We have seen already that most cases of glaucoma occur through inadequate drainage of aqueous through the drainage angle, and you may remember that we compared this to a partial obstruction of the plughole in a bath, into which water is being poured. In angle closure glaucoma, the same situation develops, but instead of a partial block, the angle becomes completely obstructed, and the situation develops suddenly, over a period of hours, rather than as a gradual change over the years. The sudden nature of the obstruction is what is referred to in the description 'acute', and this distinguishes it from the other glaucoma conditions, which sometimes are referred to as 'chronic'. Some people misinterpret the term 'chronic' to mean bad or serious, and this is incorrect – it simply means long-lasting.

The effect of a sudden, complete obstruction of the drainage angle is a rapid rise in the pressure within the eye, to a much higher level than is seen in the other types of glaucoma. Indeed, the level of pressure is high enough to lead to symptoms of pain and change in vision, which are notable for their absence in other glaucoma conditions.

The mechanism by which angle closure glaucoma develops is interesting, and important to understand in order to decide how best to treat it. Let us consider again the normal situation of aqueous production and drainage in the eye. It is produced by the ciliary body, flows through the pupil into the anterior chamber, and from here drains away into the drainage angle. In angle closure glaucoma, the flow of aqueous through the pupil is obstructed by the lens, and so the aqueous cannot drain away into the angle. Instead, it builds up behind the iris, which in turn is pushed forward, which has the effect of closing the drainage angle (see Figure 4). We can see that this very rapidly becomes a vicious circle: the more the iris is pushed forward by the build-up of aqueous behind it, the more the drainage angle will be obstructed, and the more the pressure will rise. For those of a mechanical persuasion, it might be interesting at this point to contemplate how this might best be treated, and indeed prevented from recurring. The answer is in a later section!

Who gets angle closure glaucoma?

From the above description of the mechanism of development of angle closure, it will be apparent that it is likely to develop in individuals in whom the angle between the iris and cornea is narrow in the first place, and in whom the lens either swells or is pushed forward. We know that people who are long-sighted have a much shallower chamber at the front of the eye than those who are short-sighted, and indeed angle closure is much

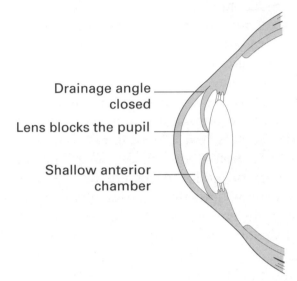

Drainage angle closed

Lens blocks the pupil

Shallow anterior chamber

Figure 4 Angle closure glaucoma

more common in long-sighted people. In addition, as we get older, it is normal for the natural lens in our eye to become fatter, and also for the supporting filaments that secure it in position to stretch somewhat. These two factors can combine to allow the lens and iris to move forward, so leading to the obstruction of the pupil that starts the process of angle closure. Those most at risk, therefore, are long-sighted individuals, as they get older.

There is also a racial predisposition to this type of glaucoma, and it is seen most commonly among the Inuit, whose risk of angle closure glaucoma is roughly 40 times greater than that of the average white population. Although it can be seen in different members of the same family, there is no strict genetic link, although the tendency to being long-sighted, which increases the risk, is often inherited.

Interestingly, the angle is most likely to obstruct when the iris is wider open, since as the pupil widens, the muscles within the iris 'ruck up' within the angle, and so obstruct it. This has the effect of making attacks of angle closure glaucoma more frequent in the winter months, when the long, dark nights tend to leave the pupil wider open for longer periods. In addition, it is quite possible for an attack to be precipitated by the drops instilled to widen the pupils during a routine eye examination.

Thankfully, this is a rare situation, since before dilating the pupils, an examiner will always inspect the angle to see if it is particularly narrow, and at risk of this development. On the rare occasions that an attack is caused by such drops, it can be readily recognized and treated. In many ways it is better for this to have been identified and dealt with, than for the person at risk to develop an attack later when not under medical supervision.

The symptoms of angle closure glaucoma

The symptoms of angle closure glaucoma are due to the sudden build-up of pressure to a very high level in the eye. While the level of pressure in the glaucomas we have discussed so far may be only modestly raised, say to 25–30mm Hg, in angle closure the pressure may reach 60mm Hg or more. At this level of pressure, there is often severe pain, but in addition there can develop a shortage of blood flow to the important structures within the eye, so as ultimately to cause damage to tissues.

The intense pressure overwhelms the ability of the cornea to pump out fluid as it should do normally, and consequently it becomes waterlogged. This in turn leads to it becoming swollen and cloudy, with consequent blurring of the vision. This disturbance in the cornea (which is not unique to glaucoma) also often scatters rays of light so as to produce a halo effect, particularly around illuminated objects. We are all familiar with the rings of light that appear around lamps on a foggy day, and this sensation may develop as an attack of angle closure glaucoma begins. The eye tends also to become very sensitive to light.

The changes in the cornea alone are sufficient to reduce the vision significantly, but the relative movement of the lens within the eye also changes its focus.

If the pressure remains high for more than a few hours, irreversible damage can be done to the nerve within the eye, while obstruction of the blood vessels can occur leading to damage to the retina or death of the muscles controlling the pupil. This compounds the difficulty in treating the condition.

The effects of the raised pressure are not confined to the eye, however, and through nerve connections from the eye, raised pressure within it can cause serious effects elsewhere in the body. In particular, it is not unusual for abdominal pain to accompany an attack, to the extent that profuse vomiting can follow. Some elderly people in particular can become very unwell through the loss of fluids and general weakness that follow such developments.

Warning attacks

An established attack of angle closure glaucoma is quite a dramatic event, and the sudden onset of severe pain and loss of vision leaves neither the person nor his or her doctor in any doubt that something is seriously wrong. It is possible, however, for mild attacks of the condition to occur, and resolve spontaneously. Under these circumstances, the same sequence of events that we have described occurs, but before the pupil becomes truly immobile, some aqueous drains away sufficiently to prevent complete closure of the angle, and the attack breaks. The effect of this is that there may be a transient rise in the pressure, sufficient to cause some swelling of the cornea and possibly some pain, which settles down spontaneously.

If an intermittent attack like this can be identified as such, and laser treatment undertaken to prevent further episodes, the risks of a more serious attack that will not break on its own can be avoided. The problem arises, however, in identifying that such mild attacks are occurring, since between attacks the pressure in the eye is likely to be completely normal, and the only identifiable hint to the diagnosis, apart from the history, is the narrowed angle on close examination of the eye. Not surprisingly, many such attacks are not diagnosed until a more serious one occurs.

The treatment of angle closure glaucoma

An established attack of angle closure glaucoma, as described above, needs urgent treatment, not only because of the severe pain that the person is experiencing, but also in order to prevent any more damage to the eye than necessary, and in particular to the optic nerve. As a general rule, the longer treatment is delayed from the onset of the attack, the more difficult it is likely to be to break the attack. The importance of early treatment cannot be overstated.

As an attack progresses, death of some of the muscle tissue within the iris occurs, making it more difficult to use drugs to constrict the pupil, which is one of the principles of management. In addition, progressive cloudiness of the cornea makes treatment more difficult, and ultimately, if the attack is not broken, the drainage angle becomes permanently damaged. The very high pressure, however, in itself prevents adequate penetration of drops applied to the eye into the inside of the eye where they can be effective.

Treatment initially, therefore, has to be given as an injection and/or tablets of a drug that stops the production of the aqueous. The drug is called *acetazolamide* or Diamox, and is usually sufficient to cause a fairly rapid, though temporary, fall in the pressure, sufficient that other drugs in the form of drops are then able to penetrate into the eye to break the attack. In our 'bath with taps on' analogy, this is the equivalent of turning off the water supply for a few hours while repairs are effected.

The goal of treatment, however, is to break the attack so that normal drainage of aqueous through the drainage angle can be restored. Reducing the pressure will certainly contribute to this, partly by allowing drops to penetrate, but also by reducing the pressure on the blood supply within the eye, so as to allow the iris muscles to work again. In order to open the now closed drainage angle, however, it is necessary to constrict the pupil, and in so doing pull open the angle, to allow fluid to drain through it once more. We can see now the reason for some urgency in the treatment. If the attack is not broken before permanent damage to the angle has occurred, even opening it again may not be sufficient to control the pressure.

The drop that is usually used to constrict the pupil is pilocarpine, which we encountered briefly earlier in the book as a rather outdated form of treatment for conventional open angle glaucoma. Though rarely used for this any more, because of its side-effects and the need for application four times a day, it is an effective drug for breaking an attack of angle closure. Once the pupil constricts, the angle can open again, and the block of the pupil by the lens is broken. The attack has then been dealt with and the eye allowed to settle down before considering measures to prevent it happening again.

Unfortunately an attack of angle closure glaucoma does not always respond readily to the treatment described above, and sometimes other drugs are necessary. If the initial dose of acetazolamide does not successfully reduce the pressure sufficiently to proceed with further treatment, it may be necessary to use an infusion of dehydrating drugs to try and 'suck out' fluid from the engorged eye. These are given through a drip infusion into the arm, and have the effect of causing a rapid dehydration of the tissues. It is a powerful way of reducing the pressure, but carries the risk of upsetting the normal metabolism of fluids in the body, particularly in those who are elderly, diabetic or suffering kidney disease. Thankfully, these difficult cases are very much the minority, and most attacks respond to simpler, less invasive remedies.

Preventing a recurrence

The treatment of an attack of angle closure glaucoma does not end here, however, since unless measures are undertaken to prevent further episodes, it is likely that the eye will be affected again, or even that the other eye may suffer similarly.

Let us return to looking at the mechanism by which an attack develops in order to consider how best to prevent such a recurrence. Initially, it is the obstruction of the pupil by the lens that prevents the normal flow of aqueous through the pupil into the front chamber of the eye, and so on into the drainage angle. By creating a small hole in the iris, such pupil block can be prevented. This is exactly what is undertaken, and these days the small hole can be created using a laser, so that any formal surgery can usually be avoided. It is sensible to treat both the affected eye and the other eye to prevent further episodes.

The laser procedure itself is quick, and not painful. First, drops are put in the eye to numb the surface, and then a small contact lens is placed on the surface of the eye, which allows the surgeon to focus the laser on the appropriate place on the iris. The hole is positioned in the peripheral part of the iris, so as to be as near to the drainage angle as possible. While the person rests his head against a chin and forehead support, the surgeon then fires a series of shots of laser, which feel like clicks occurring within the head! It normally takes only a few minutes.

Ideally, the laser treatment is undertaken as soon as possible in the unaffected eye, but it may not be possible to apply the laser to the eye suffering the attack until the cornea has cleared, which may take several days. If the cornea is clear on presentation, it may be possible to undertake the laser immediately, and indeed can be used to break the attack in the first place under ideal circumstances. The laser procedure is referred to as *peripheral laser iridotomy*.

Isaac
Isaac had never had any problems with his eyes, other than needing to wear glasses both for near and distance since the age of 15. He worked as a busy sales representative, and had noticed on two occasions in the previous six months some difficulty in driving at night on returning home from a long day at work. For a few hours he had noticed some blurring of his distance vision, and that car tail lights and traffic lights had a glow around them, at the same time as he noticed a mild ache behind his eyes. One evening, while watching the television, he noticed a much more severe pain in his right eye, and that the vision had become really blurred. Through the course of the evening this became worse, and he took some

painkillers and went to bed. Unable to sleep with the increasing pain, and beginning to feel generally unwell, he asked his wife to drive him to hospital.

He was diagnosed as suffering an acute attack of glaucoma in the right eye, and given an injection to reduce the pressure. Drops were started regularly into his eye, and he was given further pain relief. Every hour or so, somebody checked the pressure in his eyes, but it was not until early the next morning that he felt comfortable again, and his vision was still blurred. That day, he underwent laser treatment to both eyes, and he was discharged home from hospital.

The strange episodes of blurring and ache behind the eyes that Isaac experienced before the proper attack were probably mild episodes of angle closure glaucoma, which aborted spontaneously. Once the attack got a hold, however, only medical intervention was able to break it. The injection was acetazolamide, which stops production of the aqueous fluid in the eye, and the drops then could penetrate the eye to constrict the pupil and break the attack. The next day, once the cornea had cleared sufficiently to allow laser to take place, a small hole was made in the iris of each eye to prevent further attacks.

People do not always need to be admitted to hospital to treat angle closure, although many doctors prefer this, but in Isaac's case he was in severe pain, late in the night, and it was important to break the attack as soon as possible, and control his pain. Many attacks do occur late in the evening, as the pupil dilates somewhat. Once treated, Isaac never had any problems again. Thankfully, because he attended promptly, the attack broke fairly easily, and before any permanent damage had occurred.

Cataract extraction

It may seem strange to consider cataract surgery at this point, but there are occasions when the treatment of angle closure glaucoma necessitates the removal of a cataract, which is simply the cloudy lens within the eye. If we consider the mechanism of development of angle closure, it will be apparent that any enlargement of the lens of the eye, or indeed change in its shape, may potentially lead to the pupil becoming obstructed by it, and hence to the progressive sequence we discussed above. In such cases, it is necessary to remove the lens, and replace it with a plastic lens in exactly the same way as would be done with a routine cataract operation.

The difference is the difficulty and potential risks with the procedure, when the view through the cornea may be cloudy, and also the pupil will not dilate well because of the attack. For this reason, it is preferable to have the attack broken before such surgery is undertaken, if possible. There are circumstances, however, in which this is not possible, and the surgery may have to be performed under less than ideal circumstances.

Ongoing management

I referred earlier to angle closure glaucoma as being the 'appendicitis' of the eye. This may sound a strange comparison, but there are similarities between the two conditions, in that both, once treated, will not recur. It is impossible to develop appendicitis once the appendix has been removed, for obvious reasons, and equally, once successful laser has been performed, angle closure glaucoma will not recur, since the situation of pupil block cannot develop.

However, it is possible for the drainage angle to be damaged during an attack, to the extent that normal outflow of aqueous is not re-established. In this situation, even though the underlying cause of the closure of the angle may have been addressed, it remains poorly functioning. The condition then effectively becomes similar to the more conventional types of glaucoma, which we have already considered. Similarly, it may necessitate long-term treatment with drops, or even surgery. A somewhat confusing terminology is often used for this condition of chronic angle closure. Remembering that the term 'chronic' means ongoing, the term is not as confusing as it sounds, and it simply reflects the need for continued monitoring of the situation if the angle has been damaged in this way. Such damage can be assessed by the specialist inspecting it directly with the mirrored contact lens we discussed earlier.

Angle closure glaucoma is undoubtedly a more dramatic, and potentially more rapidly destructive, condition than the other forms of glaucoma we have so far considered, simply because of the dramatically high pressures that may develop. However, if diagnosed sufficiently early, and promptly treated, it can usually be rapidly brought under control, and further attacks prevented in the future. Often it is a routine examination by the optometrist that identifies the narrow angles that predispose to the condition. Once again, we see the importance of regular examinations.

9

Alternative treatments

Few diseases cure themselves, and most respond better with the active co-operation and participation of the person who has the condition. Nowhere is this more the case than in glaucoma, and it is tragic to see the few cases of blindness that could have been avoided but for neglect in either diagnosis or treatment. Helping yourself does not begin and end with taking drops as instructed, although this is crucial if they are required, but involves also an awareness of the condition such that a diagnosis can be made as early as possible, and a positive mental attitude towards its management. Quite apart from the conventional medical treatments that we have discussed already, there are other measures that can be helpful in treating glaucoma, which include alternatives or complements to conventional medical treatments, together with lifestyle and dietary considerations.

The concept of 'alternative' treatment is somewhat strained, since so many drugs used in modern medicine and regarded as quite conventional are derived from natural products anyway, and what once was alternative is often gradually accepted into routine practice. The principle of a healthy lifestyle in disease prevention and management is hardly controversial, and though again fashionable, was much more so in the days when medical treatments had so much less to offer.

The term 'alternative' implies that there is a choice to be made between conventional treatments, as recommended by the traditional medical establishment, and others proffered by practitioners outside these circles. Had some of the great pioneers and innovators of the past accepted such a rigid division between conventional and alternative medicine, we would not have seen the introduction of numerous life-saving drugs and innovations. It is interesting indeed to reflect that many of the drugs we now use routinely would not pass the stringent safety checks required of new treatments were they to be introduced in the twenty-first century. We have our ancestors to thank for the introduction of what at the time were 'alternative' treatments into the conventional medical practices of the time.

It is for this reason that I prefer the term 'complementary' treatments, since this reflects better the way that all currently available knowledge can be used to treat disease. This is not to undermine the importance of controlled research, and a logical approach to treatment, based as much as is possible on facts rather than fashion and anecdote. Let us now consider some of the treatments for glaucoma, which may complement those we have considered already.

Diet

Recent years have seen a huge growth in the recognition of the importance of diet to our health in so many respects, and in parallel the development of a huge industry offering supplements to our normal fare. Much research has been undertaken into the importance of diet in the prevention and management of many eye diseases, including glaucoma. Although there are still unanswered questions, some consistent messages have evolved, which can help in treatment.

Perhaps not surprisingly, the current main lines of research confirm what our grandparents told us many years ago: that if we eat our greens, we will live to be healthy. With regard to the eye, there is now good evidence that consuming foods rich in antioxidants is protective to the eyes. In particular, it appears that such

93

products may help in preventing the development and progression of *macular degeneration*, which is the most common condition leading to blindness in the Western world, but glaucoma too seems to benefit. Many foods contain high levels of antioxidants, but leafy green vegetables such as spinach and broccoli, as well as certain berries, and in particular bilberries, are the best sources. Omega-3 fish oils are also protective to the eyes, and can be taken either as part of a balanced diet, or as supplements.

Other research has highlighted the importance of chromium in our diet to protect against glaucoma. It appears that reduced levels may be associated with the development of raised pressure in the eye. Chromium is found in cream, full-fat milk and red meat, and, somewhat paradoxically, deliberate attempts to reduce intake of these foods by some people in search of cardiovascular health may be reducing their chromium intake.

There are hosts of dietary supplements of all types available, all claiming to protect the eyes. Before choosing to take such preparations, it is important first to consider your general diet, since often quite minor modifications, such as an increase in the consumption of green vegetables, can make significant contributions to your overall well-being, and protect your eyes as well.

If you do feel you wish to take supplements, make sure that you do not take too much: some vitamins and trace elements can be harmful in overdose, and you should not exceed the recommended intake, or take multiple preparations such that this may occur. Be careful also as to the source, since there is the risk of making an expensive – or even dangerous – purchase if buying from completely unknown suppliers. The internet is awash with offers of all kinds of preparations, so you need to be careful.

Exercise

We all know that exercise is good for us, not only for its physiological benefits, but for the psychological ones also, and the general feeling of well-being that it promotes. It is well recognized that regular exercise improves cardiovascular health, and since glaucoma is a condition associated with impaired blood supply to the optic nerve, it seems logical to expect increased fitness to be of benefit. Although it is difficult to measure precisely the effects of exercise on the development or progression of glaucoma, studies have shown that people who exercised regularly for three months reduced the pressure in their eyes by up to 20 per cent. Regular exercise goes hand in hand with sensible eating, and a healthy lifestyle. As with many conditions, it appears that such behaviour is likely to benefit glaucoma.

Smoking

The message that smoking is bad for your health is universal and beyond dispute. Even now, however, there are constant new discoveries of specific illnesses that had not previously been associated. The effects on the heart and circulation of regular smoking are well recognized, and are responsible for a large proportion of heart attacks and strokes. Knowing that glaucoma is mediated through impaired circulation to the optic nerve, it is not surprising that smoking adversely affects glaucoma, and top of the list of lifestyle changes should be stopping smoking. Although some of the complementary therapies described below have uncertain effects on glaucoma directly, when used to help you to stop smoking, they undoubtedly contribute significantly to management of the condition in a more indirect manner.

Holistic therapy

Holistic therapy basically means the management of the whole person, rather than targeting just the specific affected organ, as is generally the case with conventional medical treatment. As such, the term is used to include nutrition, exercise and methods of self-regulation such as meditation and relaxation. It is well known that such techniques and lifestyle choices can lower blood pressure, and so we could assume that glaucoma is similarly helped. The slow, insidious nature of glaucoma makes it very difficult to provide objective measures of whether any particular treatment is of benefit, and again it is difficult to be sure what contribution holistic therapy might make to any individual. The same, of course, can be said of conventional medical treatments, and we rely therefore to some extent on people's personal experiences. Anecdotal as it may be, I have a number of patients who have noted improvements following holistic therapy.

Marijuana

The smoking of marijuana is one of the more controversial treatments for glaucoma, principally since in most countries it is illegal, but also because of the adverse side-effects accompanying it. It is well known that the pressure within the eye is reduced by the use of marijuana, but unfortunately the effect is only achieved during its smoking, and is not sustained once this ceases. Attempts to use marijuana drops have been unsuccessful, and although the National Eye Institute in the USA undertook serious research into the drug, it has not transpired to be a useful aid to the management of

glaucoma. Quite apart from its mind-contorting properties, the potentially carcinogenic effects and psychological risks from its regular use have confined it to an
interesting experiment in medical history.

Acupuncture

Acupuncture has been used to treat virtually every
ailment known to mankind. Although our experience of
its use in the Western world is very modest compared to
that in China, it is becoming increasingly popular and
many qualified practitioners now operate within the UK.
So far, experiments have not proved acupuncture
capable of influencing the pressure within the eye or the
visual field, but case series have demonstrated a
subjective improvement in vision among some people.
As always with such improvements that cannot be
objectively assessed, it is difficult to know how much
these represent a placebo effect, and how much might be
genuine improvements in visual function. On the other
hand, if the treatment makes any improvement through
whatever means, it merits serious consideration anyway,
and it is for the individual to decide if it is suitable for
him or her.

Yoga

Yoga also is an import from the East that finds
increasing favour in the Western world. Few who
practise it would deny the benefits it affords in offering
mental and physical relaxation, and an increased sense
of well-being. Its use in the treatment of glaucoma
remains uncertain. The logic of undertaking anything
that can improve overall health, and in particular benefit
cardiovascular vigour, is obvious. A word of caution
regarding prolonged maintenance of a head-down or

inverted posture is worth sounding, however, since these may lead to a rise in the pressure within the eye. Like most things in life, however, it is perfectly safe in moderation.

The above comprise only a minority of the many alternative or complementary therapies available today, although most of those not listed above make no specific claims to be helpful in glaucoma, and the evidence that they are beneficial is doubtful. For the reasons I discussed above, it is best to think of them as complementary to more conventional medical treatment, rather than in competition with them. It is essential, whatever form of treatment is chosen, that the condition is monitored closely.

We have seen earlier that just starting drops is no guarantee that glaucoma will immediately be arrested, and the same applies to complementary treatments. It is only by monitoring the parameters of pressure, visual field and optic nerve head appearance that stability can be confirmed. The very insidious nature of glaucoma and its lack of symptoms until the disease is well advanced can lead to false comfort, of which both the person with the condition and the practitioner should be aware.

10
Living with glaucoma

Glaucoma is never cured, but can usually be controlled. It is encouraging to realize that 95 per cent of those diagnosed early on with glaucoma will go on to preserve their vision until the end of their natural lives, but this in most cases will require lifelong treatment with eye drops. Even if surgical or laser treatment removes this necessity, there is still a need for continued monitoring of the condition (except in some cases of angle closure glaucoma), and in this respect the condition never really completely goes away.

It is inevitable, therefore, that diagnosis, or even suspicion of the diagnosis, will have some long-lasting implications not only for you, but possibly also for your friends and family. Hopefully, these will be very modest, such as needing to instil drops regularly, and attend occasional clinic reviews for check-ups. In a small minority of people, the visual loss is sufficiently severe as to impose other restrictions, such as curtailing driving, or even becoming reliant on others for more basic needs. Whatever the level at which glaucoma affects you, the sooner you can make a positive commitment to dealing with it and any attendant lifestyle changes, the easier life is likely to be. Let us now consider in some detail exactly what living with glaucoma is likely to mean on a day-to-day basis.

Keeping up your treatment

For most people the diagnosis of glaucoma means nothing more than the regular administration of eye drops and periodic review in an eye clinic. They never develop symptoms, and their vision is well preserved indefinitely. Indeed, it is the very lack of symptoms that can make it difficult to remember, or be bothered, to keep up the treatment. Unlike many diseases, in which forgetting to take the remedy leads to rapid deterioration and an unpleasant reminder of the symptoms that prompted treatment, glaucoma gives no reminders – until it is too late. It is vital therefore to use the drops as instructed, and we discussed in Chapter 6 the merits of doing this yourself if at all possible.

It is almost inevitable that you will forget or be unable to put in your drops on the odd occasion. If this is the case, do not panic. You are unlikely to develop any severe damage through just missing the occasional drop, but remember that any damage is cumulative. If you repeatedly forget the 'occasional' drop, it is possible that you will lose vision, just as if you stopped the treatment altogether. If you cannot remember whether you have put the drops in, or if your regular schedule is delayed such that you are late in doing it, do not worry. It is better to have the drops late rather than not at all, and if you put it in twice by mistake, no harm will ensue.

When attending the eye clinic, or your optometrist, for a check-up, use the drops at the same time as you would normally do. It is most unhelpful to stop the drops on the day of examination, since if the pressure is raised, it is impossible to tell if this is because the drops are not working, or because you missed them. If you have not been taking them for any reason, it is much better to be honest with the specialist examining you rather than to pretend that you have used them, or just put them in before the visit when you have not been using them in between. If there are difficulties administering the drops, discuss it with the doctor, to see if any alternatives might be considered.

Living with a restricted field of vision

Sadly, it is not an uncommon consequence of glaucoma for the field of vision to be reduced, and this may or may not be noticeable to the person with the condition. Sometimes, if the change has been very gradual, as it often is, even quite significant loss of peripheral vision may not be recognized.

Once you become aware of loss of visual field, either yourself or because it has shown up on a field test, it is necessary to give some consideration as to how to deal with this. It may be that it troubles you only under certain conditions, such as in poor light, and if this is the case, the solution may be obvious and simple. Adequate lighting is important for us all; but particularly for those with any kind of visual impairment, it is important to ensure that there is good illumination in corridors and where stairs are present. The commonsense advice of avoiding leaving things on the stairs to trip over is particularly pertinent, since it might easily happen that such an object is within the area of missing visual field, with the obvious adverse consequences.

Generally, however, navigating about the home safely is not the main issue for those who have lost vision, since the surroundings are familiar, and the lighting controllable. In unfamiliar places, however, particularly when there is either dim or dazzling light, life can be more difficult. Resist the temptation to wear very dark glasses in an attempt to protect yourself from dazzle when outdoors. Although a tint, or lenses that react to light, may suit some, remember that in glaucoma the eye is less sensitive than normal, and if you wear deeply tinted glasses this may make your vision worse. Consider instead wearing a hat, cap or brim of whatever sort to protect you from dazzling light if this is a problem.

Awareness of the restriction in your field of vision is important, and particularly when attempting to cross the road. You should realize that while other people might pick out an approaching car in the edge of their vision, it might not be visible to you, and you will need to look around you, moving your eyes and head, much more than you have been used to. Similarly, if, say, the left half of your vision is missing, then it is sensible (and natural) to turn your head to the left somewhat to see in this area. Consider where to position yourself at social gatherings, the theatre, etc. to minimize the problems as much as you can.

Driving

In the twenty-first century we live in an age of heavy dependence on the motor vehicle, and it feels as if the whole of life is designed around the car. Those of us who drive give little attention to the difficulties experienced by those who do not, and it therefore can come as an enormous shock to lose the ability to drive. Indeed, for many people with glaucoma it is the loss of their car that is the biggest social and psychological blow: the loss of independence and feeling of dependence on others can be quite devastating, and in some cases can necessitate even moving house to be nearer to amenities, friends and relatives.

Consequently, the decision to cease driving is a big one, which sometimes is imposed by the authorities, but often is made by the person even if he or she is still within legal limits, but feels the time has come to give up. Many of those with glaucoma seem confused about the legality of driving, and before considering the other factors that influence such a decision, it is helpful to clarify the current legal position in the UK.

Driving licences are issued by the DVLA, and they

hold the responsibility for deciding whether any individual has satisfactory health, which includes vision, to drive. For this reason, part of the driving test involves a relatively crude assessment of vision whereby the candidate is asked to read a number plate at 20.5 metres. Crude though this may seem, this is the visual standard for driving a car, but in addition it is clearly important that the field of vision is not significantly impaired. The DVLA recognizes this by requiring a field of vision of 120 degrees horizontally, and at least 20 degrees both above and below the horizontal midline. It does not matter whether this is achieved with one eye, or both eyes, and many people who only have one eye fulfil this requirement.

Unfortunately, some of those with glaucoma, who have modest restriction of the field in each eye, do not have this required level of vision. It is your responsibility as a driver to inform the DVLA if you have any medical condition that might impair your ability to drive, and this obviously includes field loss through glaucoma. You may be advised to inform the DVLA by your optometrist, your specialist or your GP, but only the DVLA can make the decision as to whether you are allowed to drive. Failure to inform them is an offence, and in addition would generally invalidate your insurance policy.

When your visual field is measured in the course of monitoring glaucoma, the eyes are tested one at a time. This is important since otherwise a defect in one eye might be masked by the other eye being able to perceive stimuli within the area of loss. We discussed earlier how there is an area of overlap of visual field between the two eyes. As far as the driving requirements are concerned, however, it does not matter how the field of vision is achieved: all that is important is that the overall field is sufficient.

For this reason, you may require to have a field of vision assessment measured using both eyes. This is undertaken by an independent assessor appointed by the DVLA. Usually this is a local optometrist who has been approved as such, who will assess your visual acuity (the size of letters on the vision test chart that you can see) and measure your field of vision with both eyes open. The most common assessment of this type is called an *Esterman* test. The test is very similar to the field tests we discussed earlier, and indeed performed using the same machine, but undertaken with both eyes open. Once these assessments have been made, the DVLA will take a decision on whether you are eligible to keep your licence. In cases of doubt, where the field loss is marginal, a repeat field test may be indicated. Although the DVLA hold absolute authority to issue or revoke a licence, there is an appeal procedure through the courts – although obviously it is not wise to pursue this unless you fulfil the requirements.

The requirements for drivers of heavy goods vehicles and public service vehicles, such as lorries and buses, are more stringent, and require a better level of visual acuity.

The important point to understand is that it is the driver's responsibility to inform the DVLA of any visual impairment. Many people think that their doctor or optometrist can authorize them to drive, and this is not the case. In fact, professionals looking after you are bound by duties of confidentiality not to release information about you without your consent, and only under circumstances that would be likely to cause you to be a risk to yourself or others can this confidentiality be broken. It is obviously much more satisfactory for this situation never to arise.

The legal issue of whether you are entitled to drive is not the whole story, however. Most of us have to make a decision to stop driving at some time in our lives, however hard this may be. Vision is not the only faculty that may deteriorate as we age, and impaired hearing and slowed reflexes are common accompaniments, quite apart from a generally reduced agility that is required to take emergency action to avoid accidents. Most people can recognize that there comes a point at which they are not able to honestly say that they still have the ability to drive safely, at which point they should stop driving. Sadly, some continue, and tragedy can result, with fatal consequences either to themselves or other innocent parties.

Thankfully, the majority of people with glaucoma still fulfil driving standards, and continue to drive safely for many years, but it is an important aspect of life, and one that requires regular review. If you are in any doubt, seek the advice of your optometrist or specialist.

Glasses and other visual aids

For the majority of those with glaucoma, their spectacle requirements are not altered by the condition. One common exception to this is that people who undergo trabeculectomy surgery for the disease often need different glasses afterwards, as the change in shape of the eye modifies the lenses required. It is sensible not to seek new glasses for at least six to eight weeks after the surgery, since during this period the refraction may still be unstable. Your specialist would normally advise you about this.

Otherwise you should continue your regular visits to your optometrist as instructed. Those who wear contact lenses can continue to do so, even if using eye drops. It is best, however, to try and avoid putting drops on to your contact lenses, since build-up of the drops can damage the lenses. Try if possible to use your drops before or after you put in your lenses, at the beginning and end of the day. Increasingly, people use daily disposable contact lenses, and this avoids any problems with drops altogether.

If glaucoma becomes advanced, and particularly if it occurs in addition to other eye diseases, such as cataract or macular degeneration, it may be necessary to use other less standard forms of visual aid. These include magnifiers, which may be hand-held or rested on the document to be read, and many include their own illumination system. Other aids include telescope lenses fitted to spectacle frames. Although many optometrists stock such vision aids, some of the more specialist ones may require fitting by a specialist Low Visual Aid (LVA) clinic, usually held in a hospital.

Registering visual impairment

Although the majority of those with glaucoma will live normal lives with no restriction, some do find certain tasks difficult and others may ultimately require some support of a practical and financial nature because of their condition. In the UK, there is a system for registering visual impairment and alerting the authorities who can help. Although the mechanisms of registration have recently changed, in order to make it easier for people to refer themselves and allow high street optometrists to facilitate this as well as the more conventional registration through a hospital eye department, essentially the principle of offering support to those in need remains unchanged.

Until recently, people could be registered as 'partially sighted' or 'blind' via the BD8 form, which had to be completed by a hospital specialist. The terms were misleading, and sometimes upsetting to people, in that most of those registered 'blind' still had some useful vision, although were visually impaired sufficiently to require the same level of support as those who are completely blind. In addition, the definition of 'blind' was that it was necessary 'to be so blind as to be unable to perform any work for which eyesight is essential'. Keen scholars of English grammar will not be slow to point out the error in using the word to be defined in the definition! The terms have now been altered to 'severely sight impaired' and 'sight impaired'.

A number of mechanisms for registration exist, which include the Low Vision Leaflet, through which high street optometrists can assist people in referring themselves to the local social services for assessment, the Referral of Visual Impaired Patient, which is undertaken by hospital eye departments pending decision as to whether Certificate of Visual Impairment is issued.

The criteria for registering somebody as 'severely sight impaired' are quite strict, and somewhat technical, taking into account not only the level of acuity of the eyes (or what size of letter can be seen on the vision test chart), but also the field of vision. In glaucoma, it is usually the field of vision that is reduced rather than the acuity. It is perfectly possible to be registered as 'severely sight impaired' while still able to read quite a way down the chart, if the field is very constricted. The definition of 'sight impaired' is much looser and comprises being 'substantially and permanently handicapped by defective vision caused by congenital defect or illness or injury'. Clearly, in practice, this is open to a degree of flexible interpretation.

The benefits derived from certification are variable, dependent upon the level of certification, and the person's own circumstances, but potentially offer certain social security benefits, tax concessions and practical help within the home.

Once a social service department has received notification of somebody's certification, it is obliged to assess their needs and include their name on the local register, in order to provide help. It is important to emphasize that registration is entirely voluntary, and access to the various benefits is not dependent on registration. Having said this, there is no merit in *not* registering your visual impairment since this facilitates the processes of help to you.

Self-help groups

Self-help groups vary in structure from small, informal, local arrangements to huge international organizations, and the condition of glaucoma is well served by a number of excellent support networks. Some people like the personal support and companionship that local groups can offer, whether these exist in isolation or are affiliated to a larger organization. Others, however, prefer the anonymity of being able to hear and read about the condition, without actively going out to meet others. For this latter group, the internet provides a wealth of information and contacts, some of which are listed in Further Information at the end of this book.

The best known of these is the hugely successful International Glaucoma Association (IGA), who operate internationally to provide information and support. Funded by voluntary donations, the IGA is a registered charity and produces a number of excellent information leaflets, which are distributed widely through hospital eye departments and other outlets. By joining the IGA, you receive regular newsletters and invitations to free meetings where expert speakers discuss glaucoma, as well as details of the local support groups.

In addition to such large organizations, there may be patient support groups organized through your own hospital unit, and many areas have societies catering for the needs of visually impaired people who have lost their eyesight through whatever cause. Indeed, for some people, attending and participating in some of these support groups almost becomes a full-time job, as they get more involved and help with fundraising and other events. You may not wish to become as committed as this, but just being able to talk to somebody who lives with glaucoma can be of enormous help. The inevitability of self-help groups is that there is always somebody worse off than you, and though this can be encouraging on the one hand, it can also be distressing to see somebody who is severely visually disabled if you are fearful that the same might happen to you.

The spectrum of glaucoma might be thought of as similar to a pyramid in structure, with width representing the number of those with the condition, and the height representing the severity of it. The wide base of the pyramid represents the majority of people with glaucoma, who have no symptoms at all, and who are affected only by needing to instil drops and go for check-ups. The apex of the pyramid, representing severe loss of vision, is occupied by only a small minority of people. As the pyramid ascends, there are fewer and fewer people suffering progressively more serious disease. The purpose of this analogy is to realize that it is most unlikely that you will be affected severely by the condition, assuming, of course, that you comply with your treatment.

Aids to mobility

Some people with glaucoma do eventually find their mobility restricted, either through the loss of vision alone, or in combination with other age-related problems, such as arthritis or chest and heart disease. To many, simply carrying a white cane to indicate their visual difficulties can be a great benefit. Although some worry that this might highlight their disability to muggers or malicious pranksters, this is an extremely rare occurrence, and the help in crossing roads, or finding the way, that people who would otherwise pass by will offer can be most welcome.

A number of organizations will provide such aids, and this will usually be discussed if you are registered with the local social services. In addition, a longer cane that can be used for navigation is useful to some people with severe visual restriction. It is necessary to have training in the use of these and, along with other organizations, Guide Dogs for the Blind offers this – as well, of course, as providing guide dogs to those who may benefit.

Living with glaucoma is, for most people, a minor inconvenience rather than life-changing. We have seen the very variable, and usually insidious, nature of the disease, and the wide spectrum of symptoms and treatments this may embrace. The stark reality of glaucoma is that it can never be reversed, and as such we should all be vigilant about having regular eye checks, and taking early action to have treatment if necessary.

On the other hand, there is much to be positive about. Glaucoma is rarely a blinding condition, and recent years have seen a revolution in early diagnosis and treatment to allow so many more of those with glaucoma to lead healthy, normal lives. It is a condition to respect, but not to fear.

Further information

There are many scientific publications concerning glaucoma, and the depth to which it is possible to research the condition is limited only by the time you wish to spend. Inevitably, however, much of this information is highly technical, and not easy to understand. Below are listed some suggestions for further reading and useful websites.

Further reading and websites

Books

British National Formulary (lists medications), produced by the British Medical Association and Royal Pharmaceutical Society of Great Britain, 2005.

Garway-Heath, D., *Glaucoma: A Patient's Guide.* International Glaucoma Association, 2004.

Grehn, F., *Glaucoma.* Springer-Verlag, 2004.

Kanski, J., *Clinical Ophthalmology.* Butterworth Heinemann, 2003.

Khaw, P. T., *Glaucoma in Babies and Children.* International Glaucoma Association, 2004.

Rand Allington, R., and Bruce Shields, M., and colleagues, *Shields' Textbook of Glaucoma.* Lippincott, Williams and Wilkins, 2004.

Websites

www.glaucoma.org
This is run by the Glaucoma Research Foundation, who support much of the current research into the condition. As well as being a respected research establishment, the Foundation provides much educational literature, and this website is well laid out and most useful.

www.iga.org.uk

This is the website of the International Glaucoma Association. It contains a huge amount of information about the disease, as well as information about research sponsored by the IGA. There is a good section on Frequently Asked Questions, and a very topical Newsletter.

www.guidedogs.org.uk

The Guide Dogs for the Blind charity not only trains and provides guide dogs, but is involved as well in a host of other activities to support those with impaired vision, through whatever cause, and in research into the causes of blindness. This website gives an overview of these activities.

www.healthyeyes.org

This website is also run by the Guide Dogs for the Blind, and gives much useful information about a range of eye diseases.

www.nei.nih.gov

This is the website of the National Eye Institute, which governs most research into eye disease in the USA. The site has a huge amount of information, some of it quite technical. Quite apart from the useful information within the website, it gives a glimpse into the huge resources being poured into glaucoma research.

www.nurseseyesite.nhs.uk

This website was set up and is run by a group of specialist eye nurses. Although it is principally a forum for discussion and education between nurses, it also contains much useful patient information about cataract and other eye conditions.

FURTHER INFORMATION

www.moorfields.org.uk

Moorfields Eye Hospital is the most famous eye unit in the UK, and has an excellent website which includes information about many eye conditions, including glaucoma. There are a number of useful diagrams and illustrations.

Index

INDEX

prostaglandins

macular degeneration 94
marijuana 96–7
meditation 96
memantine 54
minim 57
Mitomycin-C 67
mobility 109–10
monitoring
   ocular hypertension
   39–43

needling 66
neuroprotection 47–9, 54
non-penetrating glaucoma
   surgery 68
normal tension glaucoma
   see glaucoma
nystagmus 9, 78

ocular hypertension
   38–45
   treatment study 40–3
open angle glaucoma *see*
   glaucoma
ophthalmoscope 23
optic cup 21
optic nerve 4
   damage 7, 12
   head 20–4, 34–5

pain 13, 83–4
pigmentary glaucoma *see*
   glaucoma
pilocarpine 53, 86

preservatives in eye drops
   56–8, 74–5
pressure 2–4
   effects 4–6, 83–4
   intraocular 15
   measurement 15–20
   normal 18, 38
   very high 43–5
primary glaucoma *see*
   glaucoma
prostaglandins 51–2
   bimataprost (Lumigan)
   52
   latanoprost (Xalatan)
   52
   travoprost (Travatan)
   52
pseudoexfoliative *see*
   glaucoma

race 1, 82
registering visual
   impairment 106–8
risk factors 2

screening 30–1
secondary glaucoma *see*
   glaucoma
slit-lamp 16, 33
smoking 95
stinging 55
sympathomimetics 54
   apraclonidine 54
   brimonidine 54
   dipivefrine 54
symptoms 13–14, 83–4